AI AWARENESS SERIES

AI in Healthcare

Marina Westcott-Gray

Contents

Introduction

A radiologist in Tokyo reviews chest X-rays with the assistance of an AI system that has analyzed millions of similar images. In rural Kenya, a community health worker uses a smartphone app powered by machine learning to diagnose diabetic retinopathy, preventing blindness in patients who might never see an ophthalmologist. At a major American research hospital, oncologists design personalized cancer treatments based on AI analysis of tumor genetics, while in London, an emergency department uses predictive algorithms to anticipate patient surges hours before they occur.

These scenarios aren't glimpses of a distant future—they represent healthcare's present reality. Artificial intelligence has moved from experimental laboratories into clinical practice with remarkable speed, fundamentally altering how we diagnose disease, plan treatments, manage hospitals, and conduct medical research. The transformation touches every aspect of healthcare, from the most sophisticated quaternary care centers to basic primary care clinics in underserved communities.

This revolution arrives at a moment of unprecedented need. Global healthcare systems strain under the weight of aging populations, with the number of people over 65 expected to double by 2050. Chronic diseases consume ever-larger portions of healthcare budgets—diabetes alone affects over 500 million people worldwide and costs more than $960 billion annually. Meanwhile, the World Health Organization projects a shortage of 10 million healthcare workers by 2030, even as

Introduction

medical knowledge doubles every 73 days, making it impossible for any individual practitioner to stay fully current.

Into this perfect storm of challenges, artificial intelligence offers not a panacea but a powerful set of tools. Machine learning algorithms can process vast amounts of medical data in seconds, identifying patterns invisible to human observation. Natural language processing systems synthesize findings from thousands of research papers, bringing evidence-based medicine to the point of care. Computer vision surpasses human accuracy in detecting certain cancers, while predictive analytics forecast patient deterioration hours before traditional monitoring would trigger alarms.

Yet the integration of AI into healthcare presents unique complexities absent from other industries. When an e-commerce algorithm makes an error, a customer might receive irrelevant product recommendations. When a healthcare AI fails, lives hang in the balance. The stakes demand exceptional rigor in development, validation, and deployment. Healthcare AI must navigate stringent regulatory requirements, address profound ethical questions about bias and fairness, and maintain the trust that forms the foundation of the patient-provider relationship.

The human element remains irreplaceable. AI excels at pattern recognition and data processing, but medicine requires empathy, ethical judgment, and the ability to navigate ambiguity— quintessentially human capabilities. The most successful healthcare AI implementations augment rather than replace human intelligence, creating partnerships where technology handles routine tasks and data analysis while clinicians focus on complex decision-making and patient interaction.

This book provides a practical guide to understanding and implementing AI in healthcare settings. It addresses both the technical foundations and real-world applications of healthcare AI. We examine not just what's possible, but what's practical, ethical, and beneficial for patients and providers alike. Each chapter builds on the previous one, creating a complete picture of how AI is reshaping medicine and what this transformation means for everyone involved in healthcare delivery.

The journey ahead explores both tremendous opportunities and sobering responsibilities. As we stand at this intersection of human wisdom and artificial intelligence, the choices we make today will determine whether AI becomes a tool for democratizing healthcare access and improving outcomes for all, or another technology that widens existing disparities. The path forward requires technical expertise, ethical clarity, and above all, an unwavering commitment to the fundamental purpose of medicine: alleviating suffering and promoting human wellbeing.

Chapter 1: Introduction to AI Technologies

Artificial intelligence represents the culmination of decades of research aimed at creating machines that can simulate human cognitive processes. The field originated from early theoretical explorations in computational theory and machine intelligence, pioneered by visionaries like Alan Turing and John McCarthy. AI has evolved through multiple phases, from symbolic AI and expert systems in the 1960s-80s, through machine learning breakthroughs in the 1990s-2000s, to today's deep learning revolution. This evolution reflects our growing understanding of how to create systems that can learn from data, recognize patterns, solve complex problems, and make intelligent decisions across diverse domains.

AI encompasses three main categories that form the foundation of modern intelligent systems. Symbolic AI uses rules and logic to represent knowledge and make inferences. Machine learning enables systems to learn patterns from data without explicit programming. Neural networks, inspired by biological brain structures, process information through interconnected nodes. Major breakthroughs include expert systems that captured human expertise in knowledge bases, deep learning advances that revolutionized pattern recognition through multi-layered neural networks, and reinforcement learning successes that enabled AI to master complex games and optimize strategies through trial-and-error interactions with environments.

Current AI trends focus on making systems more transparent, ethical, and human-centered. Explainable AI addresses the "black box" problem by making AI decision-making processes interpretable and trustworthy for users. AI ethics has become paramount, emphasizing responsible development, fairness, privacy protection, and bias mitigation across all AI applications. Increasing automation continues to transform industries, with AI enabling more processes to operate autonomously while boosting efficiency. Looking ahead, future AI systems will be more autonomous, adaptive, and designed around human needs, creating seamless human-AI collaboration across all sectors of society and industry.

Machine learning encompasses three fundamental paradigms that define how systems learn from data. Supervised learning uses labeled training data to teach models to make accurate predictions or classifications on new, unseen data. This approach powers applications like email spam detection and medical diagnosis. Unsupervised learning discovers hidden patterns and structures in unlabeled data, enabling tasks like customer segmentation and anomaly detection. Reinforcement learning takes a different approach, where agents learn optimal behaviors through trial and error, receiving rewards or penalties based on their actions. This paradigm has achieved remarkable success in game-playing AI and autonomous systems.

Deep learning architectures represent the cutting edge of artificial neural networks, enabling unprecedented capabilities in pattern recognition and data analysis. Layered neural networks form the foundation, using multiple hidden layers to model increasingly complex patterns and representations in data. Convolutional Neural Networks (CNNs) revolutionized computer vision by automatically learning spatial hierarchies and features in images, making them ideal for tasks like object recognition and medical imaging. Recurrent Neural Networks (RNNs) excel at processing sequential data such as text, speech, and time series, maintaining context and memory across time steps to understand temporal patterns and dependencies.

Machine learning and deep learning have found transformative applications across numerous industries, demonstrating their practical value in solving real-world problems. Recommendation systems power personalized experiences on platforms like Netflix and Amazon, analyzing user behavior to suggest relevant content and products. Fraud detection systems use deep learning to identify suspicious patterns in financial transactions, protecting billions of dollars annually. Autonomous vehicles represent perhaps the most ambitious application, using machine learning algorithms to perceive environments, make driving decisions, and navigate safely. Healthcare diagnostics benefit from AI's ability to analyze medical images and patient data, often achieving accuracy levels that match or exceed human specialists.

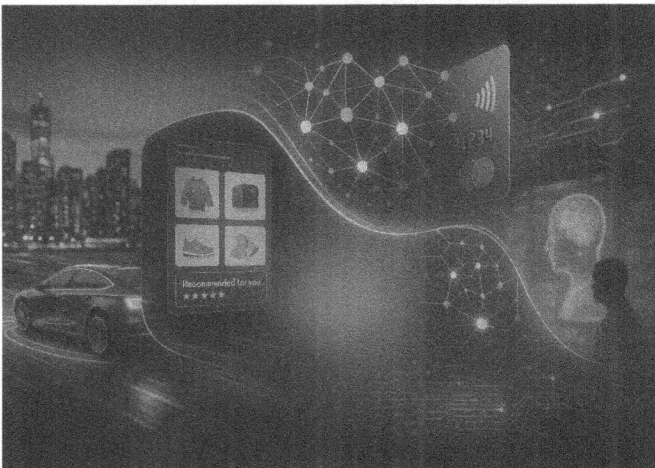

Chapter 1: Introduction to AI Technologies

Natural Language Processing rests on three fundamental linguistic concepts that enable computers to understand human language. Syntax governs the structural rules for arranging words and phrases into grammatically correct sentences, providing the foundation for language parsing and generation. Semantics focuses on meaning, helping systems understand what words, phrases, and sentences actually convey in different contexts. Pragmatics adds the crucial layer of contextual interpretation, enabling AI to understand implied meanings, cultural references, and situational nuances. Together, these three pillars allow NLP systems to process language with increasing sophistication, moving beyond simple keyword matching to genuine language comprehension and generation.

Text processing and sentiment analysis rely on several key techniques that transform raw text into structured, analyzable data. Tokenization serves as the foundation, breaking continuous text into discrete units like words or phrases for computational processing. Part-of-speech tagging assigns grammatical categories to each word, enabling deeper syntactic analysis. Named Entity Recognition identifies and classifies important entities such as people, organizations, locations, and dates within text. Sentiment analysis represents the culmination of these techniques, gauging opinions, emotions, and attitudes expressed in textual content. These techniques work together to enable sophisticated text understanding and automated content analysis across diverse applications.

NLP applications have transformed how we interact with technology and process information at scale. Chatbots for customer service demonstrate NLP's ability to understand customer inquiries and provide real-time, contextually appropriate responses, reducing response times and operational costs. Machine translation tools like Google Translate leverage advanced NLP to convert text between languages instantly and with increasing accuracy, breaking down communication barriers globally. Automated content generation represents an emerging frontier, where NLP systems create summaries, articles, and reports, dramatically improving content production efficiency while maintaining quality and relevance across diverse domains and industries.

Computer vision's core capabilities center on teaching machines to interpret and understand visual information with human-like accuracy. Image recognition assigns specific labels to images by analyzing their visual content, enabling applications from photo organization to quality control in manufacturing. Image classification organizes visual data into predefined categories using sophisticated algorithms, particularly Convolutional Neural Networks that have revolutionized the field. CNNs represent the technological breakthrough that made modern computer vision possible, using specialized architectures that automatically learn hierarchical features and patterns from visual data, achieving unprecedented accuracy in tasks ranging from medical imaging to autonomous navigation.

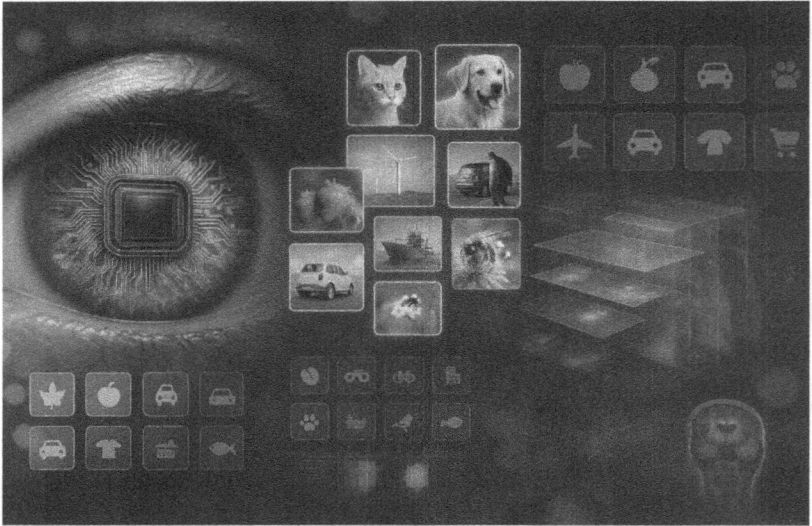

Advanced computer vision techniques enable machines to understand complex visual scenes with remarkable precision. Object detection goes beyond simple classification to identify and locate multiple objects within images, drawing bounding boxes around items and providing their precise coordinates. Image segmentation divides images into meaningful regions or segments, enabling detailed analysis of specific areas and pixel-level understanding of visual content. Motion tracking extends these capabilities to video streams, following object trajectories across frames to monitor movement patterns. These techniques combine to create comprehensive visual understanding systems used in surveillance, autonomous vehicles, sports analysis, and medical imaging applications.

Computer vision's practical applications demonstrate its transformative impact across critical industries. Medical imaging diagnostics leverage computer vision to enhance accuracy in analyzing X-rays, MRIs, and

CT scans, often detecting abnormalities that human radiologists might miss while reducing diagnosis time. Autonomous vehicles rely heavily on computer vision to perceive their environment, identifying roads, obstacles, pedestrians, and traffic signals to navigate safely without human intervention. Surveillance and threat detection systems use computer vision for security applications, automatically identifying suspicious activities, unauthorized access, and potential threats in real-time, providing enhanced safety and security across public and private spaces.

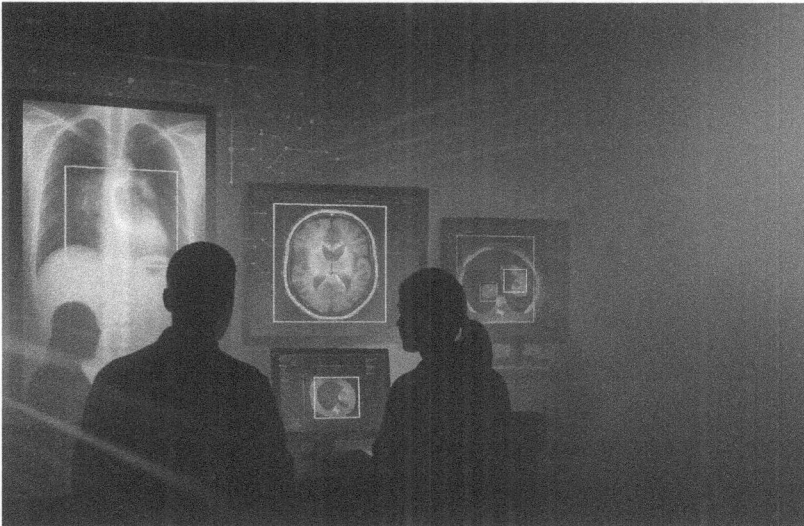

Generative models represent a revolutionary approach to AI that creates new content rather than simply analyzing existing data. Generative Adversarial Networks (GANs) use an innovative competitive architecture where two neural networks—a generator and discriminator—compete against each other, with the generator learning to create increasingly realistic synthetic data by trying to fool the discriminator. Variational Autoencoders (VAEs) take a different approach, learning the underlying probability distributions of data through encoding and decoding processes, enabling them to generate new samples that maintain the statistical properties of the training data. Both architectures have opened new frontiers in creative AI applications.

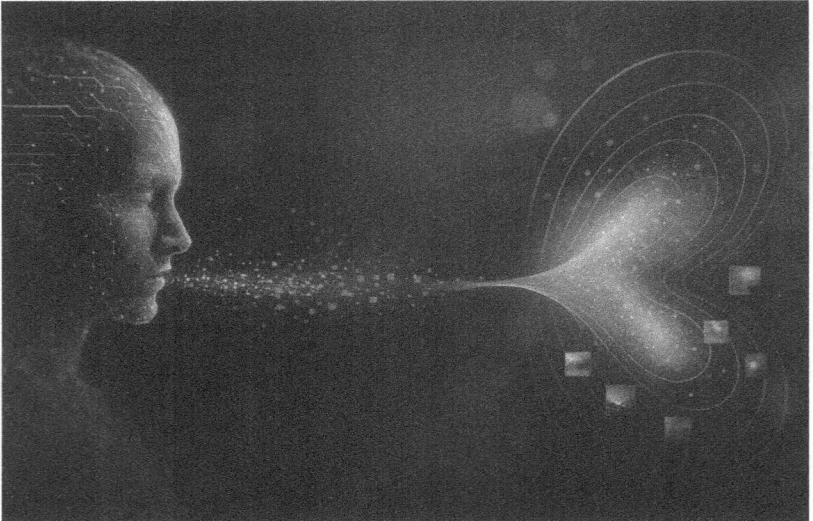

Large Language Models represent the pinnacle of natural language AI, built on transformer architecture that has revolutionized how machines process and generate human language. Transformer architecture uses attention mechanisms to efficiently process vast amounts of text data, enabling models to understand context and relationships between words across long sequences. These models' text processing capabilities stem from training on massive text corpora, allowing them to generate coherent, contextually appropriate language outputs that can engage in conversations, answer questions, write articles, and perform complex language tasks. The scale and sophistication of these models continue to grow, pushing the boundaries of what's possible in AI-human interaction.

Generative AI has opened unprecedented creative and practical possibilities across content creation and design industries. Content creation has been revolutionized, with AI enabling automated and efficient production of articles, marketing copy, social media posts, and multimedia content across various platforms and formats. Design automation leverages AI to streamline creative processes, automatically generating graphics, layouts, logos, and visual elements with increasing speed and precision while maintaining professional quality standards. Art generation represents perhaps the most visible application, with AI producing unique artworks, illustrations, and creative pieces that expand possibilities for artists and designers. These tools enhance human creativity by providing inspiration, generating variations, and automating routine tasks.

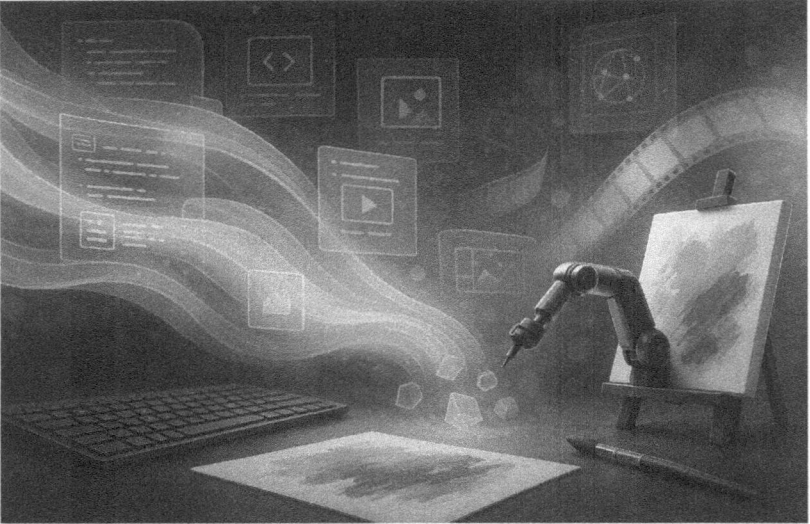

Edge computing fundamentally changes how we process and analyze data by bringing computation closer to where data is generated. Local data processing eliminates the need to send all information to centralized data centers, instead processing it on devices at the network's edge, reducing bandwidth requirements and infrastructure costs. Reduced latency is perhaps the most significant advantage, enabling real-time responses critical for applications like autonomous vehicles, industrial automation, and augmented reality experiences. Efficient AI decision-making becomes possible when processing occurs near data sources, allowing for immediate responses to changing conditions while reducing network traffic and improving overall system performance and reliability.

The integration of AI into IoT devices creates intelligent systems that can operate autonomously and respond to changing conditions in real-time. AI-enhanced automation enables IoT devices to perform complex tasks in smart homes and industrial settings, automatically adjusting heating, lighting, and security systems while optimizing energy usage and improving user convenience. Real-time monitoring capabilities allow AI-powered IoT devices to continuously assess environmental conditions, equipment performance, and system health, providing immediate alerts and responses in applications ranging from smart cities to factory automation. Intelligent edge processing allows these devices to make decisions locally, reducing dependence on cloud connectivity while enhancing privacy and system reliability.

Real-time intelligence faces significant challenges while simultaneously offering tremendous opportunities for innovation. Device resource limitations present ongoing challenges, as edge devices often have constrained processing power and memory, requiring careful optimization of AI algorithms for efficient operation. Security risks pose another significant concern, with distributed edge devices creating multiple potential attack vectors that require robust protection mechanisms and secure communication protocols. However, improved responsiveness offers major opportunities, enabling faster decision-making and immediate system reactions that can transform industries. Scalability and privacy represent additional opportunities, with edge architectures enabling secure, distributed intelligence that can grow organically while preserving user privacy and data sovereignty.

Core AI technologies—machine learning, natural language processing, computer vision, and generative models—are revolutionizing industries from healthcare and finance to entertainment and manufacturing. Emerging trends like edge AI and IoT integration are driving smarter, more efficient applications that operate in real-time, bringing intelligence directly to where it's needed most. The future impact of AI promises enhanced intelligence, improved efficiency, and broad transformation across all sectors of society. As these technologies continue to evolve and converge, they will create unprecedented opportunities for innovation, productivity, and human-AI collaboration.

Chapter 2: Data in Healthcare AI

Electronic Health Records and Data Standards represent the foundational infrastructure of modern healthcare data management. This section explores how standardized digital systems enable seamless information exchange while supporting AI development and clinical decision-making across healthcare organizations.

Overview of Electronic Health Records

Electronic Health Records revolutionize healthcare by digitizing patient information for enhanced accessibility and clinical decision support. EHRs transform traditional paper records into searchable, shareable digital formats that healthcare providers can access instantly from any location. This digital transformation improves care coordination, reduces medical errors, and enables comprehensive patient tracking across multiple healthcare encounters. The structured nature of EHRs facilitates data analysis and supports evidence-based medicine, making them invaluable for both clinical practice and AI model development in healthcare settings.

Key Data Standards in Healthcare (HL7, FHIR, DICOM)

Healthcare data standards ensure consistent information exchange across diverse systems and organizations. HL7 provides the foundational framework for sharing clinical and administrative data between different healthcare applications. FHIR represents the next evolution, utilizing modern web technologies and APIs to enable more flexible, real-time data exchange. DICOM specifically addresses medical imaging needs, ensuring that radiological images and associated metadata can be consistently stored, transmitted, and interpreted across different imaging systems and healthcare providers, supporting AI applications in medical imaging.

Interoperability and Integration Challenges

Healthcare systems face significant challenges in achieving seamless data integration due to diverse platforms and inconsistent data quality. Multiple vendors, legacy systems, and varying implementation standards create complex integration scenarios that require careful planning and technical expertise. Data quality variations across systems can lead to incomplete patient records, duplicate entries, and inconsistent formatting that hampers effective AI model training. These challenges necessitate robust data governance frameworks, standardized APIs, and comprehensive data validation processes to ensure reliable information exchange and maintain system interoperability.

Data Privacy and Compliance represents one of the most critical aspects of healthcare AI development. This section examines the regulatory frameworks that govern healthcare data protection and their implications for AI system design and deployment.

Overview of HIPAA and GDPR Regulations

HIPAA and GDPR establish comprehensive frameworks for protecting sensitive health information in their respective jurisdictions. HIPAA focuses specifically on healthcare data privacy and security requirements in the United States, mandating strict controls over protected health information access and disclosure. GDPR provides broader data protection rights for EU residents, including healthcare data, with emphasis on individual consent and data subject rights. Both regulations require healthcare organizations and AI developers to implement robust security measures, obtain appropriate consent, maintain audit trails, and ensure data is processed lawfully and transparently.

Implications for AI Development and Deployment

Healthcare AI systems must be designed with privacy and regulatory compliance as core requirements rather than afterthoughts. Regulatory compliance demands implementing privacy-by-design principles, ensuring that data protection measures are integrated throughout the AI development lifecycle. Secure data handling requires encryption, access controls, and audit logging to prevent unauthorized access and maintain data integrity. These requirements influence AI architecture decisions, data processing methods, and model training approaches, often necessitating techniques like differential privacy, secure multi-party computation, or federated learning to maintain compliance while enabling effective AI development.

Ethical Considerations and Best Practices

Ethical AI deployment in healthcare requires transparency, informed consent, accountability, and fairness throughout the development and implementation process. Transparency involves clearly communicating how AI systems make decisions and what data is used, building trust with patients and healthcare providers. Obtaining proper informed consent ensures patients understand how their data will be used in AI applications. Accountability measures establish clear responsibility chains for AI decisions and outcomes. Fairness and equity considerations require ongoing monitoring to prevent discriminatory outcomes and ensure AI systems serve all patient populations equitably, regardless of demographics or socioeconomic status.

Structured vs Unstructured Health Data represents a fundamental distinction in healthcare information systems. This section explores the characteristics, challenges, and opportunities presented by different data types in healthcare AI applications.

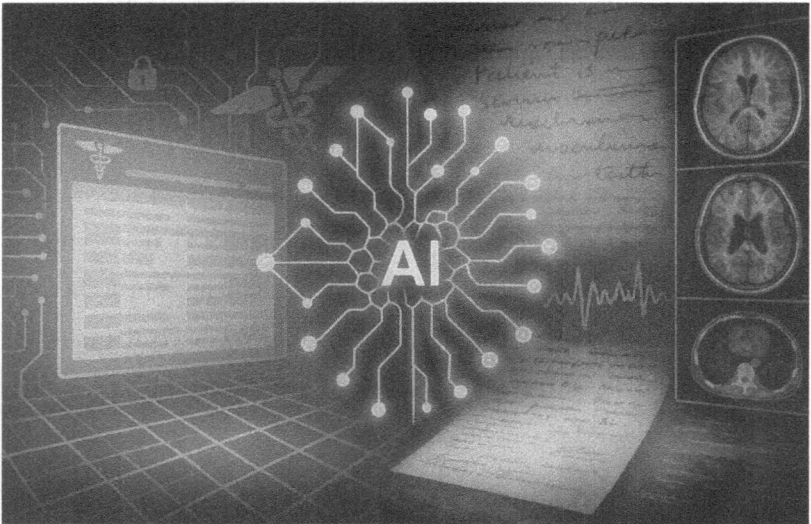

Definition and Examples of Structured Data

Structured healthcare data follows predefined formats and schemas, making it easily searchable, analyzable, and processable by computer systems. Examples include laboratory results with specific value ranges, demographic information in standardized fields, diagnostic codes using systems like ICD-10, and medication dosages with standard units. This data type enables straightforward statistical analysis, trend identification, and machine learning model training. Structured data's organized nature facilitates automated processing, quality checks, and integration across different healthcare systems, making it particularly valuable for predictive analytics and clinical decision support systems.

Definition and Examples of Unstructured Data

Unstructured healthcare data lacks predefined organization, requiring advanced processing techniques to extract meaningful information. Clinical notes represent the largest source of unstructured data, containing detailed patient observations, treatment plans, and physician insights in free-text format. Medical images including X-rays, MRIs, and CT scans require computer vision techniques for analysis. Audio recordings from patient consultations or dictated reports need natural language processing for interpretation. This data type often contains rich contextual information not captured in structured formats, making it valuable for comprehensive patient understanding and AI model enhancement.

Challenges in Processing and Integrating Both Data Types

Integrating structured and unstructured healthcare data presents significant technical and organizational challenges. Data format diversity requires different processing approaches, storage systems, and analysis techniques for each data type. Integration complexity increases exponentially when combining multiple data sources with varying structures, quality levels, and update frequencies. Advanced AI methods including natural language processing, computer vision, and multimodal learning are necessary to effectively process and unify diverse data formats. Successful integration requires sophisticated data pipelines, standardized preprocessing workflows, and robust quality assurance processes to ensure meaningful insights.

Data Quality, Bias, and Fairness constitute critical considerations for developing effective and equitable healthcare AI systems. This section addresses the challenges and solutions for ensuring AI systems provide fair and accurate healthcare outcomes.

Importance of Data Quality in Healthcare AI

High-quality data forms the foundation for reliable healthcare AI systems that can safely support clinical decision-making. Accurate data ensures AI predictions and recommendations reflect true patient conditions rather than data collection errors or inconsistencies. Complete datasets prevent gaps that could lead to misdiagnosis or inappropriate treatment recommendations. Representative data ensures AI models perform effectively across diverse patient populations, geographic regions, and healthcare settings. Poor data quality can result in biased predictions, reduced model performance, and potentially harmful clinical recommendations, making data quality assessment and improvement essential for healthcare AI success.

Detecting and Mitigating Bias

Healthcare data bias can perpetuate and amplify existing healthcare disparities, making bias detection and mitigation crucial for equitable AI systems. Bias impacts manifest in differential diagnosis accuracy, treatment recommendations, and resource allocation across patient groups. Detection techniques include statistical analysis of model performance across demographic groups, fairness metrics evaluation, and systematic data auditing to identify underrepresented populations. Mitigation strategies involve diversifying training datasets, implementing algorithmic fairness constraints, using bias-aware machine learning techniques, and conducting ongoing monitoring to ensure equitable outcomes across all patient populations served by the AI system.

Ensuring Fairness and Equitable Outcomes

Fair AI systems require intentional design and ongoing monitoring to deliver unbiased healthcare across all patient populations. Developing fair systems involves diverse training data, bias-aware algorithms, and regular performance auditing across demographic groups. Equitable patient outcomes require continuous assessment of AI recommendations to ensure no systematic disadvantages for specific populations. This includes monitoring for disparities in diagnostic accuracy, treatment recommendations, and resource allocation. Achieving fairness requires interdisciplinary collaboration between AI developers, healthcare providers, ethicists, and community representatives to identify potential bias sources and implement effective mitigation strategies throughout the AI lifecycle.

Federated Learning and Secure Data Sharing represent innovative approaches to healthcare AI collaboration that preserve privacy while enabling broader data utilization. This section explores these emerging technologies and their transformative potential for healthcare AI development.

Introduction to Federated Learning

Federated learning revolutionizes healthcare AI by enabling collaborative model training without centralizing sensitive patient data. Decentralized processing allows multiple healthcare organizations to contribute to AI model development while keeping data within their secure environments. Enhanced privacy protection results from data never leaving its origin institution, reducing privacy risks and simplifying compliance with regulations like HIPAA and GDPR. Leveraging diverse datasets from multiple institutions improves model robustness and generalizability across different patient populations, healthcare practices, and geographic regions, ultimately leading to more effective and widely applicable healthcare AI solutions.

Benefits and Limitations of Secure Data Sharing

Secure data sharing offers significant advantages while presenting notable implementation challenges. Improved collaboration enables researchers and healthcare providers to leverage collective knowledge and datasets for better AI model development and clinical insights. However, technical complexity requires sophisticated encryption, secure communication protocols, and advanced infrastructure that demand specialized expertise and significant resources. Regulatory barriers create additional challenges, as different jurisdictions have varying data protection requirements that must be carefully navigated. Organizations must balance the benefits of collaboration against implementation costs, technical requirements, and regulatory compliance obligations when considering secure data sharing initiatives.

Real-World Applications and Emerging Trends

Federated learning applications in healthcare are expanding rapidly, demonstrating practical benefits for AI advancement while maintaining privacy protection. Healthcare AI advancement through federated approaches enables development of more robust diagnostic tools, treatment recommendation systems, and predictive models that benefit from diverse institutional datasets. Compliance and privacy advantages make federated learning particularly attractive for healthcare organizations concerned about data sharing regulations and patient privacy. Emerging trends include cross-institutional research collaborations, multi-hospital AI model training, and global health initiatives that leverage federated learning to address healthcare challenges while respecting local data governance requirements and cultural considerations.

Conclusion

Data forms the essential foundation for all healthcare AI innovations, requiring careful attention to quality, bias, and privacy considerations. Privacy considerations remain paramount when handling sensitive healthcare information, necessitating robust security measures and regulatory compliance. High-quality diverse data types improve AI accuracy and reliability, supporting better clinical outcomes. Innovative data sharing methods like federated learning enable broader collaboration while preserving patient privacy, opening new possibilities for healthcare AI advancement and global health improvements.

Chapter 3: AI in Diagnostics

Artificial intelligence in diagnostics represents a paradigm shift from traditional reactive medicine to proactive, data-driven healthcare. AI systems leverage sophisticated algorithms to process vast amounts of medical data, including imaging studies, laboratory results, genetic information, and patient histories. These systems excel at pattern recognition, identifying subtle abnormalities that might escape human detection. The clinical decision support aspect is particularly valuable, as AI provides consistent, evidence-based recommendations that can reduce diagnostic variability. This technology doesn't replace clinical judgment but enhances it, offering physicians a powerful tool to improve diagnostic accuracy while reducing the cognitive load associated with complex medical decision-making.

The implementation of AI in healthcare diagnostics offers transformative benefits across multiple dimensions. Enhanced diagnostic accuracy stems from AI's ability to analyze complex datasets without fatigue or cognitive biases that can affect human interpretation. Error reduction is achieved through consistent application of diagnostic criteria and flagging of potential oversights. The speed advantage is particularly crucial in emergency situations where rapid diagnosis can be life-saving. Perhaps most importantly, AI enables truly personalized medicine by analyzing individual patient data to recommend tailored treatment approaches. These systems can identify subtle patterns in patient data that correlate with treatment responses, enabling precision medicine approaches that optimize outcomes for each individual patient.

Despite its promise, AI adoption in healthcare faces significant hurdles that must be addressed for successful implementation. Data quality remains paramount, as AI systems are only as reliable as the data they're trained on. Incomplete, biased, or inconsistent datasets can lead to flawed diagnostic recommendations. Algorithm transparency is crucial for building physician trust and meeting regulatory requirements. Many AI systems operate as "black boxes," making it difficult to understand how they reach specific conclusions. Workflow integration presents practical challenges, requiring significant changes to established clinical processes. Ethical concerns around bias, privacy, and accountability require careful consideration. Regulatory frameworks must evolve to ensure patient safety while enabling innovation in this rapidly advancing field.

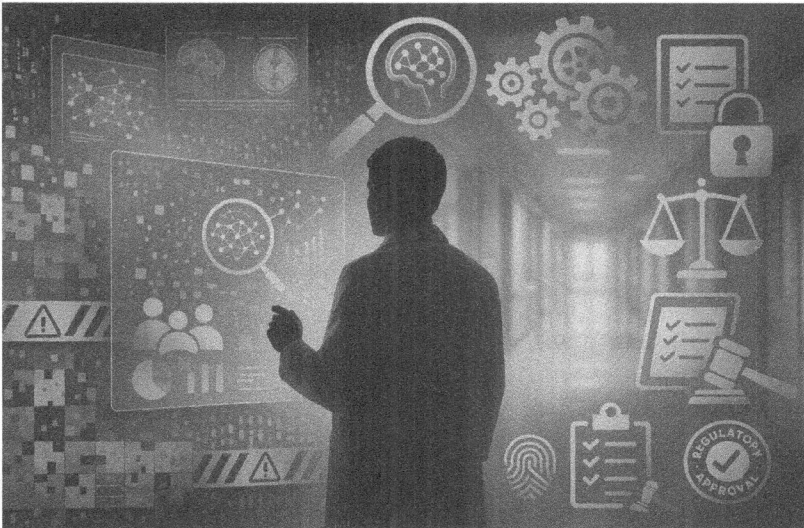

Medical imaging represents one of AI's most successful applications in healthcare, with algorithms demonstrating remarkable proficiency in detecting abnormalities across various imaging modalities. These systems excel at analyzing radiological images, including X-rays, CT scans, MRIs, and ultrasounds, often identifying subtle patterns invisible to the human eye. AI algorithms can detect early-stage cancers, fractures, neurological abnormalities, and cardiovascular conditions with impressive accuracy. The technology serves as an invaluable second opinion for radiologists, flagging potentially concerning findings and reducing the likelihood of missed diagnoses. This collaborative approach between AI and human expertise has proven particularly effective in improving diagnostic confidence and reducing interpretation errors in complex cases.

AI implementation in radiology workflows addresses critical operational challenges while improving patient care quality. Urgent case prioritization ensures that critical findings receive immediate attention, potentially saving lives in emergency situations. The reduction in interpretation times allows radiologists to focus on complex cases requiring human expertise while AI handles routine screenings. This efficiency gain is particularly valuable given the global shortage of radiologists and increasing imaging volumes. Error minimization occurs through consistent application of diagnostic criteria and systematic analysis of imaging data. These improvements translate into faster patient care, reduced healthcare costs, and better resource utilization. The technology also supports continuous learning, with AI systems improving their performance as they process more cases.

Real-world implementations of AI in radiology demonstrate measurable improvements across multiple healthcare metrics.

Chapter 3: AI in Diagnostics

Healthcare institutions report significant increases in diagnostic accuracy rates, particularly for conditions like lung cancer, breast cancer, and stroke detection. The technology has proven especially valuable in settings with limited radiologist availability, such as rural hospitals and emergency departments. Operational efficiency improvements include reduced turnaround times for imaging reports, decreased workload for radiologists, and improved patient satisfaction scores. These case studies also reveal important lessons about implementation challenges, including the need for comprehensive staff training, robust data governance, and careful algorithm validation. Success stories highlight the importance of viewing AI as a collaborative tool rather than a replacement for human expertise.

Digital pathology combined with AI represents a revolutionary advancement in disease diagnosis and treatment planning. AI algorithms analyze digitized tissue slides with unprecedented precision, identifying cellular patterns, morphological features, and molecular markers that inform diagnostic decisions. These systems excel at quantifying biomarkers, providing objective measurements that reduce inter-observer variability in pathology interpretation. Disease pattern detection capabilities extend beyond human visual capacity, identifying subtle changes in tissue architecture that may indicate early disease stages or predict treatment responses. The integration of AI in pathology workflows enables faster turnaround times for biopsy results while maintaining or improving diagnostic accuracy, ultimately accelerating patient care and treatment initiation.

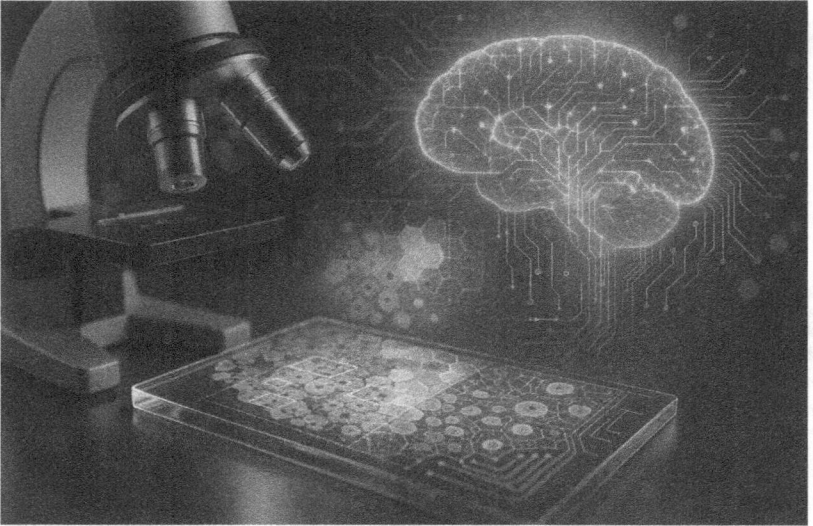

Automation in pathology addresses critical workforce challenges while enhancing diagnostic reliability. By reducing repetitive tasks and standardizing analyses, AI minimizes errors caused by fatigue, time pressure, or subjective interpretation variations. This technology allows pathologists to focus their expertise on complex cases requiring human judgment and experience. Workload pressure alleviation is particularly important given the global shortage of pathologists and increasing demand for diagnostic services. AI systems can handle routine screenings, preliminary assessments, and quantitative analyses, freeing pathologists to concentrate on challenging cases, research activities, and direct patient consultation. This redistribution of responsibilities improves job satisfaction among pathologists while ensuring optimal use of their specialized skills and knowledge.

Integration with laboratory information systems creates a seamless diagnostic ecosystem that optimizes data flow and clinical decision-making. Efficient data management ensures accurate tracking of specimens, automated quality control, and real-time updates to clinical teams. Enhanced workflow coordination eliminates bottlenecks in the diagnostic process, reducing delays that can impact patient care. The system automatically flags urgent cases, prioritizes workloads, and ensures consistent communication between laboratory and clinical staff. Comprehensive diagnostic reporting provides clinicians with detailed, standardized information that supports evidence-based treatment decisions. This integration also enables quality assurance monitoring, outcome tracking, and continuous improvement of diagnostic processes. The result is a more efficient, accurate, and responsive pathology service that better serves patient needs.

Machine learning applications in disease prediction represent a paradigm shift toward preventive and precision medicine. These systems analyze vast datasets encompassing patient demographics, medical history, laboratory results, imaging studies, and even genetic information to identify individuals at risk for specific conditions. The algorithms excel at detecting subtle patterns and correlations that may not be apparent to human clinicians, enabling early intervention strategies that can prevent disease development or progression. Predictive models for conditions like diabetes, cardiovascular disease, and cancer have shown remarkable accuracy in clinical studies. This proactive approach to healthcare has the potential to reduce healthcare costs, improve patient outcomes, and shift medical practice from reactive treatment to preventive care strategies.

Risk stratification models powered by AI provide clinicians with powerful tools for patient management and resource allocation. These systems generate personalized risk scores that help prioritize patient care, ensuring that high-risk individuals receive appropriate attention and interventions. The algorithms consider multiple risk factors simultaneously, creating comprehensive profiles that inform treatment decisions. Customized treatment plans emerge from these risk assessments, enabling precision medicine approaches tailored to individual patient characteristics and risk profiles. Effective resource allocation based on risk stratification ensures optimal use of healthcare resources, directing intensive interventions toward patients most likely to benefit. This systematic approach to patient management improves outcomes while controlling costs and enhancing the overall efficiency of healthcare delivery systems.

Ethical considerations and data privacy concerns are paramount in predictive diagnostics implementation. Informed consent processes must clearly explain how AI systems use patient data and what insights may be generated. Patients need to understand the implications of predictive analytics and maintain control over their health information. Data security measures must protect sensitive patient information from unauthorized access, breaches, or misuse. This includes robust encryption, access controls, and audit trails. Bias mitigation strategies are essential to ensure fair and equitable predictions across diverse patient populations. Algorithm developers must actively address potential biases in training data and model outputs. Patient confidentiality must be maintained throughout the diagnostic process, with clear policies governing data sharing, storage, and use for research purposes.

Chapter 3: AI in Diagnostics

Clinical decision support systems powered by AI enhance diagnostic accuracy by providing evidence-based recommendations and comprehensive differential diagnoses. These systems integrate patient data with vast medical knowledge databases to suggest potential diagnoses and treatment options. The technology excels at flagging rare conditions that might be overlooked and ensuring that all relevant diagnostic possibilities are considered. Evidence-based recommendations draw from current medical literature, clinical guidelines, and best practice protocols, ensuring that clinical decisions are grounded in the latest scientific evidence. The system serves as an intelligent assistant, augmenting clinical expertise rather than replacing it. This collaboration between human judgment and artificial intelligence leads to more thorough diagnostic evaluations and improved patient care outcomes.

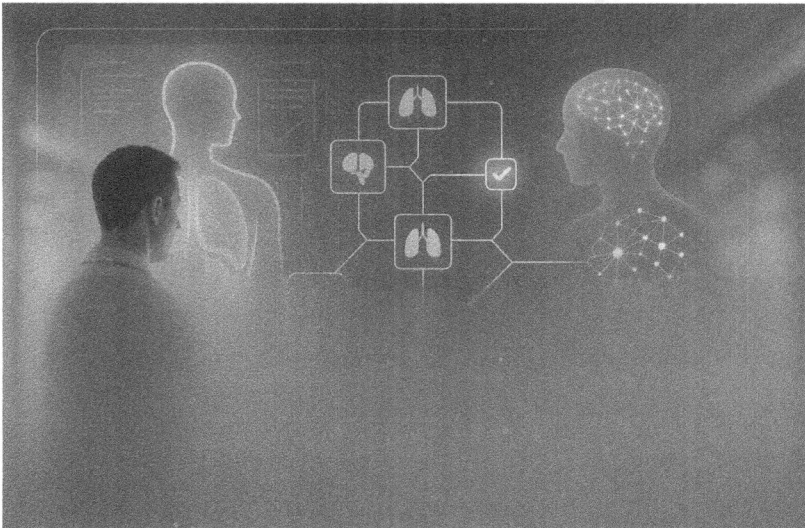

Chapter 3: AI in Diagnostics

AI's capability in complex case analysis is particularly valuable for rare disease detection and challenging diagnostic scenarios. These systems excel at identifying atypical presentations and connecting seemingly unrelated symptoms to underlying conditions. Advanced algorithms analyze vast amounts of clinical data to identify patterns that may not be immediately apparent to human clinicians. This enhanced diagnostic confidence comes from the system's ability to consider multiple variables simultaneously and compare findings against extensive medical databases. The technology is especially valuable in cases where time is critical or when dealing with conditions outside a clinician's primary area of expertise. AI-driven insights contribute to more accurate diagnoses and appropriate treatment plans, ultimately improving patient care quality and outcomes.

Current limitations in AI diagnostics include data quality issues, regulatory hurdles, and the need for extensive validation across diverse patient populations. Algorithm performance can vary significantly based on the quality and representativeness of training data. Regulatory frameworks are still evolving, creating uncertainty about approval processes and compliance requirements. Clinician training represents a critical success factor, requiring comprehensive education programs to ensure effective AI tool utilization. Healthcare professionals need to understand both the capabilities and limitations of AI systems. Future developments will focus on improving algorithm explainability, enabling seamless integration with clinical workflows, and fostering enhanced collaboration between AI systems and healthcare providers. These advancements will address current limitations while expanding AI's diagnostic capabilities and clinical utility.

Chapter 3: AI in Diagnostics

In conclusion, artificial intelligence is fundamentally transforming medical diagnostics across all healthcare specialties. The technology enhances diagnostic accuracy through sophisticated pattern recognition and data analysis capabilities that complement human expertise. Improved patient outcomes result from earlier disease detection, more accurate diagnoses, and personalized treatment approaches enabled by AI insights. However, successful implementation requires careful navigation of technical, ethical, and regulatory challenges. Healthcare organizations must invest in robust data governance, comprehensive staff training, and thoughtful integration strategies. The future of healthcare diagnostics lies in the synergistic collaboration between artificial intelligence and human clinical expertise, promising a new era of precision medicine and improved patient care. This transformation represents not just technological advancement, but a fundamental evolution in how we approach disease prevention, diagnosis, and treatment.

Chapter 4: AI in Treatment Planning and Precision Medicine

We begin our exploration with the foundational concepts of AI in treatment planning and precision medicine. This section establishes the groundwork for understanding how artificial intelligence transforms healthcare delivery through personalized approaches. We'll examine the core technologies, methodologies, and applications that enable healthcare providers to move beyond one-size-fits-all treatments toward individualized care plans. These AI-driven approaches leverage patient-specific data to optimize treatment decisions, improve outcomes, and reduce adverse effects through intelligent analysis and predictive modeling capabilities.

AI applications in personalized healthcare center on three key areas that revolutionize patient care delivery. Predictive analytics uses machine learning to analyze patient data patterns, identifying risk factors and forecasting disease progression before symptoms appear. This enables proactive interventions and preventive care strategies. Decision support systems provide clinicians with real-time, evidence-based recommendations during patient encounters, improving diagnostic accuracy and treatment selection. Automated treatment recommendations analyze complex patient profiles including medical history, genetic factors, and current conditions to suggest optimal therapy options tailored to individual patient characteristics and needs.

Several key technologies enable effective AI-driven treatment planning in modern healthcare settings. Machine learning algorithms process vast amounts of patient data to identify patterns and improve treatment accuracy through continuous learning from outcomes. Natural language processing allows AI systems to interpret unstructured clinical notes, research papers, and medical literature, extracting relevant insights for treatment decisions. Big data analytics aggregates information from electronic health records, medical imaging, laboratory results, and patient monitoring devices. Data integration combines these diverse sources to create comprehensive patient profiles that enhance AI's ability to predict treatment responses and optimize therapeutic approaches.

Precision medicine faces several challenges while offering significant opportunities for improved patient care. Data quality remains a critical concern, as AI systems require accurate, complete, and standardized information to generate reliable recommendations. Inconsistent data formats, missing information, or measurement errors can compromise AI performance. Privacy and transparency issues involve protecting sensitive patient information while maintaining algorithmic transparency for clinical trust. However, opportunities include enhanced diagnostic accuracy through pattern recognition, optimized treatment selection based on individual patient characteristics, and real-time monitoring capabilities that enable dynamic treatment adjustments for improved outcomes and reduced adverse effects.

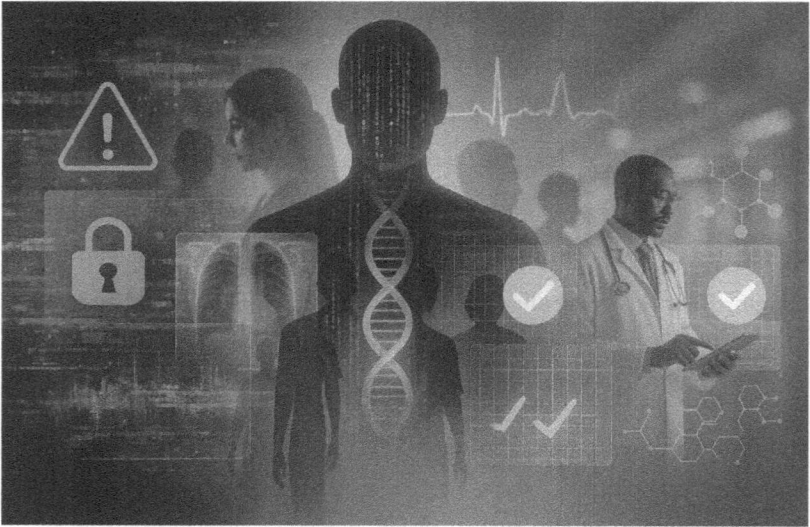

Oncology represents one of the most promising areas for AI application in treatment optimization. Cancer care involves complex decision-making processes that benefit significantly from AI's ability to analyze multiple data sources simultaneously. This section explores how artificial intelligence enhances cancer diagnosis, staging, treatment selection, and monitoring throughout the patient journey. AI applications in oncology leverage imaging analysis, genomic data, treatment response patterns, and clinical outcomes to provide more precise, personalized cancer care that improves survival rates and quality of life for patients.

AI algorithms significantly enhance cancer diagnosis and staging through three primary approaches. AI imaging analysis processes medical images including CT scans, MRIs, and pathology slides with greater accuracy and speed than traditional methods, detecting subtle abnormalities that human observers might miss. Pattern recognition capabilities identify early-stage cancers by analyzing tissue characteristics, cellular structures, and morphological features that indicate malignancy. AI tools assist medical professionals by providing radiologists and pathologists with consistent, rapid evaluations for cancer staging, reducing diagnostic variability and enabling faster treatment initiation. These systems serve as valuable second opinions, improving diagnostic confidence and accuracy.

Machine learning revolutionizes personalized therapy selection through data-driven approaches that consider individual patient characteristics. Data-driven therapy recommendations analyze complex patient information including tumor genetics, biomarkers, medical history, and treatment responses to suggest optimal therapy combinations. This approach moves beyond standard protocols toward individualized treatment strategies. Optimizing treatment effectiveness involves targeting tumors more precisely while minimizing side effects through better drug selection and dosing. Predictive response modeling uses historical data and patient-specific factors to forecast how individuals will respond to different treatments, enabling clinicians to select therapies with highest success probability and avoid ineffective options.

Adaptive treatment monitoring represents a significant advancement in cancer care through continuous assessment and real-time adjustments. Dynamic patient monitoring uses AI tools to track treatment responses, side effects, and disease progression throughout therapy, providing continuous feedback on treatment effectiveness. Outcome prediction leverages predictive models to forecast treatment results, helping clinicians anticipate complications and adjust strategies

38

proactively. Real-time therapy adaptation allows clinicians to modify treatment plans based on ongoing AI analysis of patient responses, optimizing therapeutic approaches as conditions change. This dynamic approach improves treatment success rates while minimizing unnecessary toxicity and adverse effects.

Genomics and AI-driven therapies represent the forefront of precision medicine, where genetic information guides treatment decisions. This section examines how artificial intelligence processes complex genomic data to identify therapeutic targets and develop personalized treatment approaches. AI applications in genomics enable analysis of vast genetic datasets, identification of disease-causing mutations, and development of targeted therapies based on individual genetic profiles. These advances are transforming treatment approaches across multiple disease areas, particularly cancer, rare genetic disorders, and complex chronic conditions requiring personalized therapeutic interventions.

AI-powered genomic data analysis transforms our understanding of disease mechanisms through sophisticated computational approaches. Advanced AI algorithms process enormous genomic datasets, identifying significant patterns, mutations, and genetic variations that contribute to disease development and progression. These systems analyze thousands of genetic markers simultaneously, detecting subtle associations that traditional analysis methods might miss. Understanding disease mechanisms becomes more precise as AI interprets complex genetic interactions, regulatory networks, and pathway disruptions. Therapeutic target discovery accelerates through AI identification of potential drug targets, enabling development of new treatments that address specific genetic abnormalities underlying individual patient conditions.

Identifying mutations and actionable targets forms the foundation of personalized genomic medicine through AI-enhanced analysis. AI systems excel at mutation detection, analyzing genetic sequences to identify critical alterations that influence disease progression and treatment response. These tools distinguish between benign variations and pathogenic mutations with high accuracy. Biomarker identification enables development of targeted therapies by pinpointing genetic signatures that predict treatment response. AI analyzes correlations between genetic profiles and therapeutic outcomes to identify actionable targets. Precision medicine benefits emerge as targeted therapies focus on individual genetic profiles, improving treatment effectiveness while reducing adverse effects through personalized approaches tailored to each patient's unique genetic makeup.

Designing personalized medicine based on genetic profiles represents the ultimate goal of genomic AI applications in healthcare. Genomic insights integration involves AI systems processing comprehensive genetic information alongside clinical data to understand individual patient profiles completely. This holistic approach considers genetic variations, expression patterns, and regulatory mechanisms that influence treatment responses. Customized treatment regimens emerge from this analysis, with AI recommending specific therapies, dosages, and combinations based on genetic compatibility. These personalized approaches improve treatment outcomes by matching therapies to individual genetic characteristics while reducing side effects through better drug selection and dosing strategies tailored to genetic metabolism and response patterns.

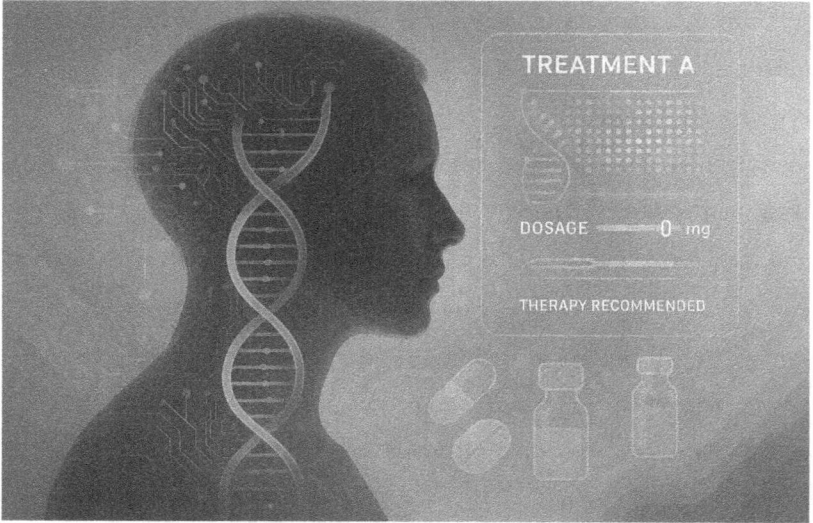

AI applications in surgery and robotics are revolutionizing surgical practice through enhanced precision, improved outcomes, and reduced complications. This section explores how artificial intelligence and robotic systems work together to transform surgical procedures across medical specialties. From preoperative planning to intraoperative guidance and postoperative monitoring, AI-enhanced surgical systems provide surgeons with advanced tools for better patient care. These technologies enable minimally invasive approaches, improve surgical accuracy, and support complex procedures that were previously challenging or impossible to perform safely.

Robotic-assisted surgical systems enhance surgical capabilities through three key advantages that improve patient outcomes. Enhanced surgical dexterity provides surgeons with greater precision and control during complex procedures through robotic instruments that eliminate hand tremor and enable precise movements in confined spaces. Improved visualization offers high-definition 3D imaging that surpasses human visual capabilities, allowing surgeons to see fine anatomical details with enhanced clarity and depth perception. Minimally invasive techniques become possible through robotic assistance, enabling smaller incisions that reduce patient trauma, minimize scarring, decrease infection risk, and accelerate recovery times compared to traditional open surgical approaches.

AI applications in surgical planning and intraoperative guidance provide surgeons with intelligent support throughout procedures. Preoperative anatomical modeling uses AI algorithms to create detailed, patient-specific 3D models from medical imaging data, enabling surgeons to plan optimal approaches, identify potential challenges, and rehearse complex procedures before entering the operating room. Real-time surgical guidance during procedures provides AI-powered navigation, tissue recognition, and decision support that enhances surgical accuracy while minimizing risks. These systems analyze live surgical data, compare it to preoperative plans, and alert surgeons to potential complications or deviations, enabling immediate corrective actions for optimal outcomes.

Outcome improvement and risk reduction through automation represents a significant advancement in surgical safety and effectiveness. Automation in surgery involves AI-controlled systems performing routine tasks with consistent accuracy, reducing human error during repetitive or precision-critical aspects of procedures. These automated functions include suturing, cutting, and tissue manipulation with programmed precision. Data-driven decision support enhances clinical decision-making through real-time analysis of surgical parameters, patient vital signs, and procedural outcomes. AI systems continuously monitor surgical progress, predict potential complications, and recommend interventions to improve patient safety and treatment outcomes throughout the surgical experience.

Digital twin models for patient simulation represent an emerging frontier in personalized healthcare, creating virtual representations of individual patients for treatment optimization. This section explores how digital twins integrate real-time patient data with physiological modeling to enable virtual testing of treatments before implementation. These sophisticated simulations allow healthcare providers to predict treatment outcomes, optimize therapy plans, and minimize risks through virtual experimentation. Digital twin technology promises to revolutionize healthcare delivery by enabling truly personalized medicine through individualized patient modeling and simulation capabilities.

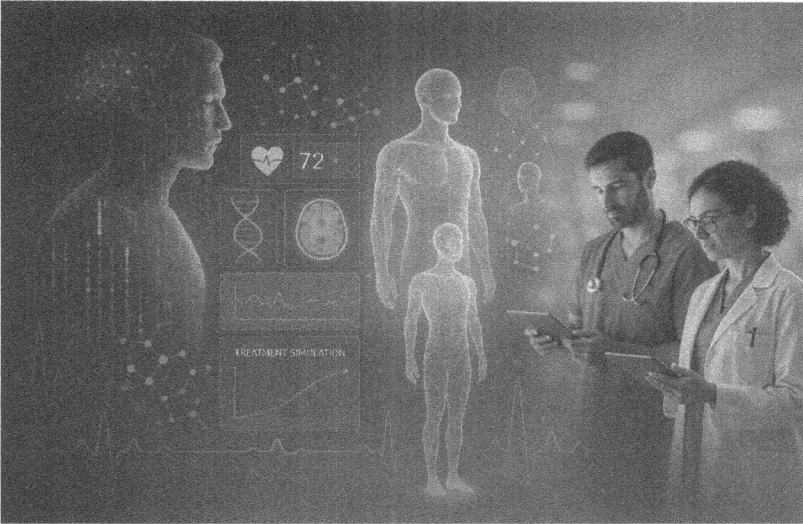

Digital twins in healthcare comprise three essential components that enable comprehensive patient modeling and simulation. Integration of patient data involves continuously collecting and processing real-time information from electronic health records, medical devices, wearable sensors, and diagnostic tests to maintain accurate patient representations. Physiological modeling creates sophisticated simulations of body functions, organ systems, and disease processes that predict health outcomes and support medical decision-making. Artificial intelligence in simulation enhances digital twins through advanced analytics that analyze data patterns, forecast future health states, and optimize treatment recommendations based on individual patient characteristics and responses to various therapeutic interventions.

Patient-specific treatment simulation enables virtual testing and optimization of therapeutic approaches before implementation. Virtual testing of treatments allows clinicians to simulate various treatment strategies safely, evaluating potential outcomes without risk to actual patients. This capability enables comparison of different therapeutic options to identify optimal approaches. Optimization of therapy plans occurs through predictive simulations that forecast treatment effectiveness, side effects, and long-term outcomes before actual implementation, reducing uncertainties and improving treatment selection. Risk minimization uses patient-specific models to identify potential complications and adjust treatment plans based on virtual results, enabling safer therapeutic approaches tailored to individual patient characteristics and risk factors.

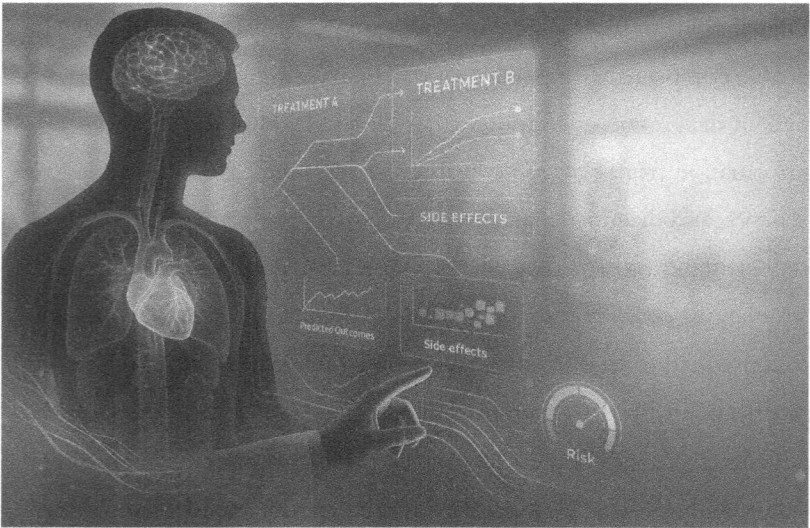

Digital twin technology benefits and future directions promise continued advancement in personalized healthcare delivery. Personalized care benefits include tailored treatment solutions that improve patient outcomes through real-time monitoring, predictive analytics, and individualized treatment optimization based on continuous data integration. Cost reduction advantages emerge through early problem identification, treatment optimization, and reduced complications that decrease overall healthcare expenses. Future integration with wearables will enable continuous health data collection for more accurate and responsive digital twin models. Advanced AI analytics will enhance predictive accuracy and decision-making support, making digital twins increasingly valuable tools for precision medicine and personalized healthcare delivery.

AI in treatment planning enables personalized healthcare through intelligent analysis of patient data, creating tailored treatment approaches that improve outcomes while reducing adverse effects. Machine learning algorithms continuously learn from treatment results to refine recommendations and optimize therapeutic strategies. Precision medicine advancements leverage AI's ability to analyze complex datasets including genetic information, medical history, and real-time health monitoring to develop highly individualized treatment plans. Innovation and collaboration in AI healthcare continue advancing through partnerships between technology companies, healthcare providers, and research institutions, driving development of more sophisticated tools that enhance patient outcomes and improve healthcare system efficiency across all medical specialties.

Chapter 5: AI in Patient Monitoring

AI applications in healthcare monitoring encompass three fundamental pillars that are reshaping patient care delivery. Data collection involves AI systems continuously gathering real-time patient health data from diverse monitoring devices, creating comprehensive datasets for analysis. Predictive analytics represents the core intelligence layer, where AI algorithms process this collected data to predict potential health issues before they become critical, enabling proactive rather than reactive care. Decision support completes the cycle by providing clinicians with data-driven insights and evidence-based recommendations that improve both patient care quality and safety outcomes throughout the treatment process.

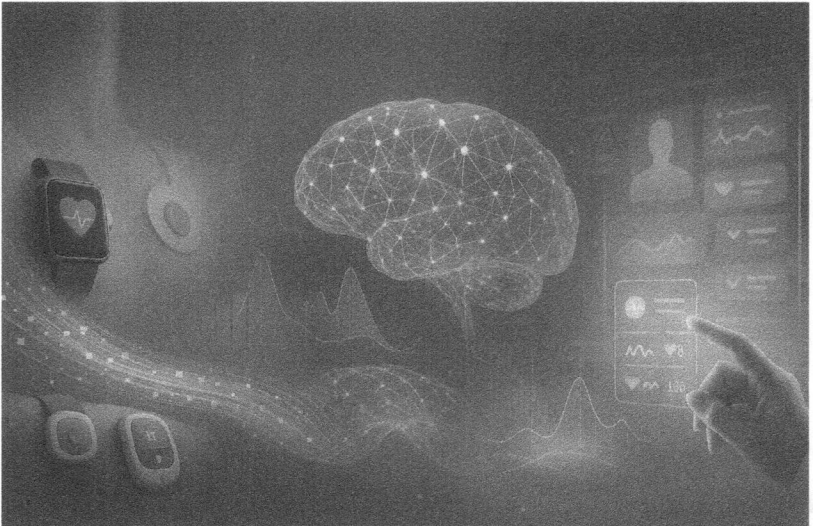

AI-driven patient monitoring delivers significant benefits while presenting important implementation challenges. The improved accuracy and early detection capabilities enhance diagnostic precision and enable healthcare providers to identify patient complications before they escalate. Personalized patient care becomes possible through AI's ability to tailor treatment plans to individual patient needs and specific medical conditions. However, data privacy and security remain critical challenges, requiring robust protection of sensitive patient information. Additionally, workflow integration challenges persist as healthcare organizations work to seamlessly incorporate AI systems into existing clinical processes without disrupting established care delivery patterns.

Four key technologies serve as the foundation for AI implementation in patient care systems. Machine learning algorithms analyze vast amounts of patient data to predict clinical outcomes and optimize treatment plans with unprecedented efficiency and accuracy. Natural language processing enables AI systems to understand and interpret complex medical records and patient communications, extracting meaningful insights from unstructured healthcare data. Advanced sensor technologies provide continuous, real-time monitoring of patient vital signs, creating comprehensive data streams that enhance personalized care delivery. Cloud computing infrastructure supports secure storage and rapid access to large volumes of patient health data, enabling scalable AI applications across healthcare networks.

Two primary categories of wearable devices are transforming health data collection in remote monitoring applications. Smartwatches and fitness trackers represent the consumer-grade category, monitoring essential metrics like activity levels, heart rate patterns, and sleep quality to promote overall health awareness among users. These devices make continuous health monitoring accessible to the general population. Specialized medical devices constitute the professional-grade category, featuring advanced sensors that measure biochemical markers and comprehensive vital signs for continuous medical monitoring. These sophisticated devices enable healthcare providers to remotely track patients with chronic conditions or those requiring intensive monitoring outside traditional clinical settings.

AI plays three crucial roles in interpreting the vast amounts of data generated by wearable devices. Data pattern recognition involves AI algorithms processing large volumes of wearable-generated data to identify meaningful health patterns and trends that might be invisible to human analysis. This capability transforms raw sensor data into actionable health intelligence. Anomaly detection enables AI systems to identify unusual health signals and deviations from normal patterns, triggering alerts for potential health issues that require early medical intervention. Actionable health insights represent the ultimate goal, where AI provides both clinicians and patients with specific, evidence-based recommendations to proactively manage health conditions and optimize wellness outcomes.

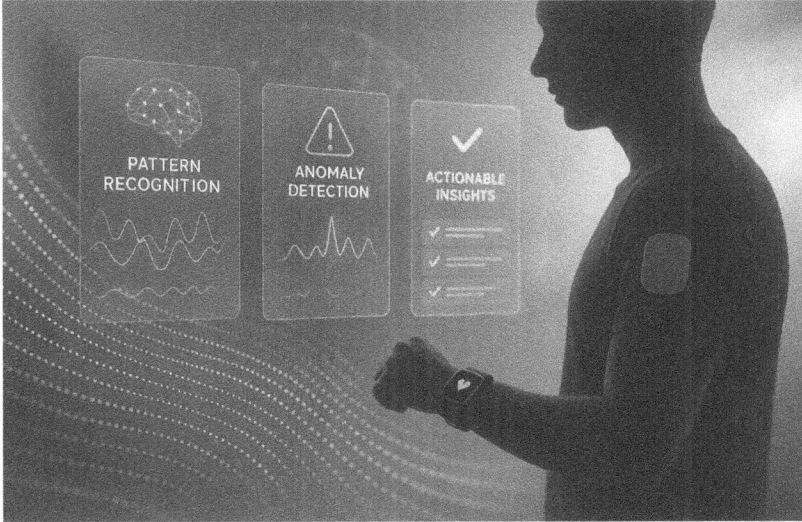

Remote monitoring technologies significantly impact patient engagement and chronic disease management through two primary mechanisms. Enhanced patient involvement occurs when AI-powered remote monitoring tools provide patients with real-time health feedback and personalized care insights, creating a more active partnership between patients and their healthcare providers. This continuous feedback loop encourages patients to take greater responsibility for their health outcomes. Chronic disease management benefits substantially from remote monitoring capabilities that enable healthcare providers to deliver timely interventions and develop truly personalized treatment plans based on continuous data streams, improving long-term health outcomes for patients with conditions requiring ongoing medical attention.

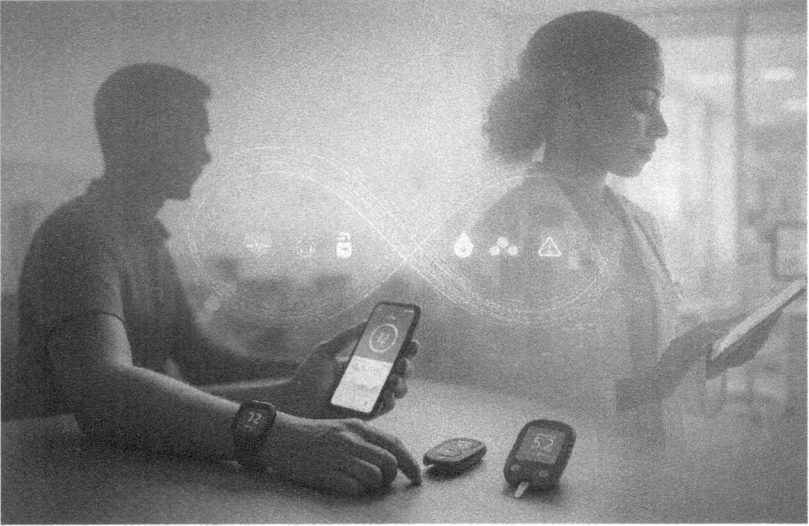

AI systems for continuous ICU monitoring operate through three integrated functions that enhance critical care delivery. Real-time data processing involves AI systems continuously analyzing physiological data streams from ICU patients, detecting critical changes in patient status with speed and accuracy that surpasses traditional monitoring methods. Alert generation represents the communication layer, where AI generates timely, prioritized alerts to notify medical staff about potential patient safety risks in intensive care units, reducing response times to critical events. Clinical decision support completes the system by providing clinicians with data-driven insights and evidence-based recommendations that improve patient care decisions in high-stakes ICU environments where split-second decisions can impact patient survival.

Patient deterioration detection and rapid response capabilities represent critical advantages of AI implementation in intensive care settings. Early detection with AI enables algorithms to identify patient decline patterns earlier than traditional clinical observation methods, providing healthcare teams with extended intervention windows that can be crucial for patient outcomes. This predictive capability transforms reactive care into proactive medical management. Rapid clinical intervention becomes possible when early identification systems enable faster, more targeted medical responses to emerging health crises. This shortened response time significantly reduces the likelihood of adverse outcomes in critical care environments, where timing often determines the difference between recovery and serious complications or mortality.

Integration with hospital information systems creates three essential capabilities that enhance overall healthcare delivery. Seamless AI integration ensures smooth data flow between AI monitoring systems and existing hospital infrastructure, creating enhanced clinical workflows that support rather than disrupt established care processes. Unified data access combines Electronic Health Records with AI-generated insights, providing healthcare teams with comprehensive, real-time access to patient information that supports better clinical decision-making. Workflow enhancement represents the practical benefit of integration, where automated AI systems reduce manual tasks, minimize human errors, and streamline administrative processes, allowing healthcare providers to focus more attention on direct patient care rather than data management and documentation tasks.

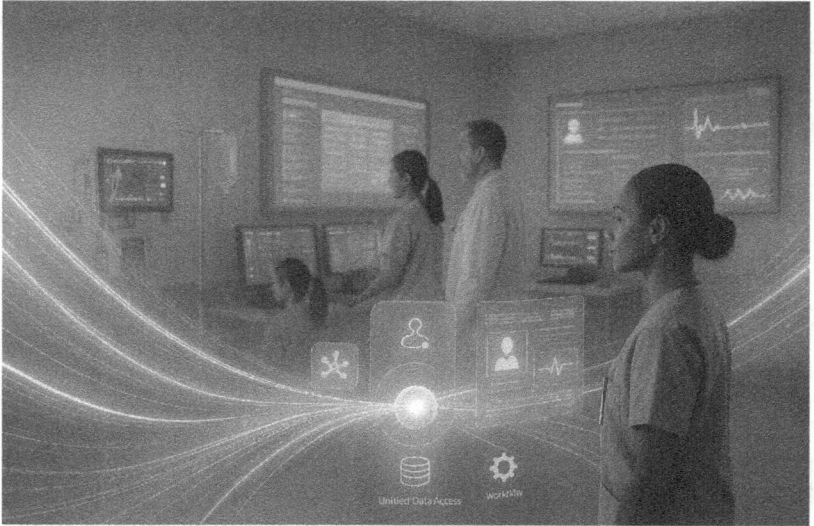

AI algorithms for predicting adverse events operate through three interconnected mechanisms that revolutionize preventive healthcare. Machine learning applications in healthcare enable AI models to process complex, multi-dimensional patient data, identifying subtle risk patterns that precede adverse events and might be missed by traditional clinical assessment methods. Predicting critical events represents the core functionality, where sophisticated algorithms forecast serious conditions including sepsis, cardiac arrest, and respiratory failure with sufficient lead time to enable effective medical intervention. Enabling preemptive care transforms healthcare delivery from reactive to proactive, as early warning systems help healthcare providers intervene before critical health events occur, fundamentally improving patient safety and clinical outcomes.

Early warning system deployment demonstrates measurable improvements across three key performance indicators in healthcare settings. AI adoption in hospitals has led to widespread implementation of AI-based early warning systems that significantly enhance patient monitoring capabilities and enable more timely medical interventions. Improved detection rates represent quantifiable benefits, as AI systems consistently demonstrate increased accuracy in identifying patients at risk for critical events, enabling faster and more appropriate clinical responses to emerging health threats. Reduced mortality outcomes provide the most significant validation of these systems, with clinical data showing that timely AI-generated alerts contribute directly to lower mortality rates in hospital environments, demonstrating the life-saving potential of artificial intelligence in healthcare.

Clinical outcomes and case studies demonstrate three significant improvements resulting from AI early warning system implementation. Enhanced clinical decision-making occurs as AI systems provide healthcare providers with comprehensive, data-driven insights that support more timely and accurate clinical decisions, reducing diagnostic uncertainty and improving care coordination. Reduced ICU stays represent both clinical and economic benefits, as AI-driven early intervention capabilities have led to measurably decreased lengths of stay in intensive care units, indicating faster patient recovery and more efficient resource utilization. Improved survival rates provide the most compelling evidence of AI effectiveness, with documented cases showing that AI-driven early warning systems contribute to higher patient survival rates in critical care environments, validating the transformative impact of artificial intelligence on healthcare outcomes.

Chapter 5: AI in Patient Monitoring

Automated tracking and interpretation of vital signs encompasses three integrated AI capabilities that transform patient monitoring. Continuous vital signs monitoring enables AI systems to track essential physiological parameters including heart rate, blood pressure, and oxygen saturation levels in real-time, providing comprehensive patient assessment without gaps in coverage. Accurate data interpretation represents the analytical power of AI, where sophisticated algorithms analyze vital sign data to detect early signs of abnormalities and identify critical health conditions before they become clinically apparent through traditional observation methods. Clinician alert systems complete the monitoring cycle by automatically notifying healthcare providers about abnormal vital sign readings, ensuring timely medical intervention when patient status changes require immediate clinical attention.

Machine learning models for risk assessment operate through four key functions that optimize healthcare resource allocation and patient care. Patient data evaluation involves comprehensive analysis of diverse patient information, including medical history, current vital signs, laboratory results, and demographic factors to create accurate health risk profiles. Risk stratification enables these models to categorize patients by risk levels, allowing healthcare teams to prioritize clinical attention and allocate resources effectively based on patient need severity. Guiding interventions ensures that risk assessments translate into proactive, tailored medical interventions that address individual patient needs. Resource allocation optimization helps healthcare organizations focus their limited resources on patients with the greatest clinical needs, improving overall care efficiency and patient outcomes.

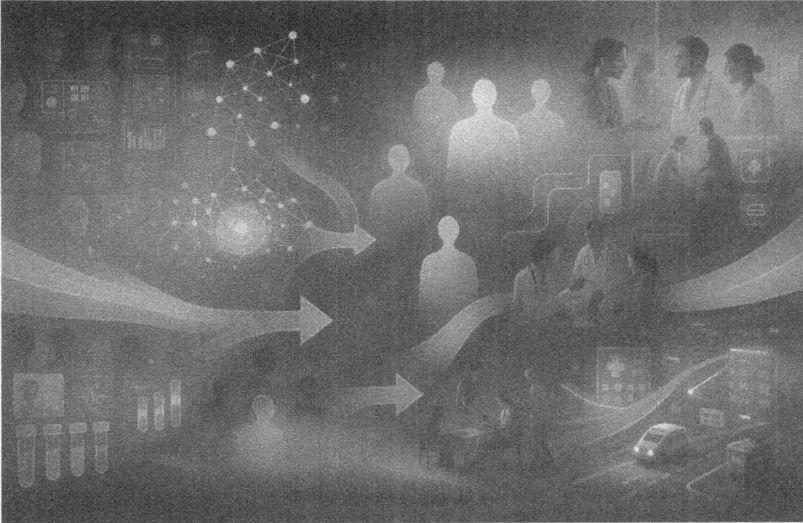

Personalization of care through AI insights operates through two fundamental processes that enhance treatment effectiveness. Integration of patient data involves AI systems combining comprehensive patient information including medical history, current vital signs, laboratory results, and other relevant health data to create detailed, individualized health profiles that guide clinical decision-making. This holistic approach ensures that all aspects of a patient's health status inform care planning. Optimized treatment plans represent the practical application of AI insights, where tailored care strategies developed through artificial intelligence analysis improve treatment effectiveness and enhance overall patient outcomes by addressing individual patient characteristics, preferences, and specific medical needs rather than applying generic treatment protocols.

Our exploration of AI in patient monitoring reveals four transformative benefits that are reshaping healthcare delivery.

Chapter 5: AI in Patient Monitoring

Enhanced accuracy demonstrates how AI improves the precision of patient monitoring systems, significantly reducing diagnostic errors and increasing reliability across all aspects of healthcare delivery. Early intervention capabilities enable healthcare providers to detect health issues in their earliest stages, allowing for timely medical interventions that dramatically improve patient outcomes and reduce healthcare costs. Personalized care represents AI's ability to tailor healthcare plans to individual patient characteristics and needs, enhancing treatment effectiveness through customized monitoring and intervention strategies. Future innovation promises continued advancement, as ongoing AI developments will further transform healthcare delivery, creating new possibilities for patient care and positive health outcomes.

Chapter 6: AI in Hospital Operations

Artificial intelligence encompasses three core technologies transforming healthcare delivery. Machine learning algorithms process vast amounts of medical data to enhance diagnostic accuracy and predict patient outcomes more reliably than traditional methods. These systems continuously learn from new data, improving their performance over time. Data analytics applications enable hospitals to make evidence-based decisions by efficiently processing complex healthcare datasets, revealing patterns and trends that inform strategic planning. Automation technologies streamline routine hospital workflows, reducing manual tasks and minimizing human error. Together, these AI applications create integrated systems that enhance operational efficiency while supporting clinical decision-making. The synergy between machine learning, analytics, and automation provides hospitals with powerful tools to optimize resource allocation, improve patient care quality, and reduce operational costs.

AI implementation in hospitals delivers significant benefits while presenting manageable challenges. The primary advantages include enhanced diagnostic accuracy through pattern recognition, improved operational efficiency via automated workflows, and better patient outcomes through data-driven insights. AI systems can process information 24/7, providing consistent support for clinical and administrative decisions. However, hospitals must address several implementation challenges. Data privacy and security concerns require robust cybersecurity measures and compliance protocols. Complex system integration demands careful planning and technical expertise to ensure AI tools work seamlessly with existing hospital information systems. Comprehensive staff training is essential for successful adoption, requiring investment in education programs. Successfully balancing these benefits against implementation challenges requires strategic planning, adequate resource allocation, and strong leadership commitment to digital transformation initiatives.

AI implementation across hospitals demonstrates versatility in addressing diverse operational challenges. Patient triage systems use machine learning algorithms to quickly assess symptom severity, prioritizing emergency cases and improving response times during peak periods. This reduces wait times and ensures critical patients receive immediate attention. Predictive maintenance applications analyze equipment performance data to forecast potential failures, enabling proactive maintenance scheduling that prevents costly downtime and ensures continuous operation of critical medical devices. Resource allocation optimization systems use real-time data to distribute medical staff and equipment efficiently across departments, responding dynamically to patient volume fluctuations. Administrative task automation streamlines paperwork processing, appointment scheduling, and documentation, reducing staff workload and minimizing errors. These diverse applications showcase AI's ability to enhance both clinical and operational aspects of hospital management simultaneously.

Predictive analytics transforms patient flow management through sophisticated forecasting capabilities. AI systems analyze historical admission patterns, seasonal trends, and real-time data to accurately predict patient admissions and discharges. This data-driven forecasting improves hospital planning efficiency by enabling proactive resource allocation and staff scheduling. The system considers multiple variables including emergency department volumes, scheduled surgeries, and discharge patterns to provide comprehensive predictions. Optimized bed capacity management helps hospitals proactively address potential overcrowding situations before they occur, reducing patient wait times and improving satisfaction. AI forecasting enables better staffing plans by predicting when additional healthcare personnel will be needed, ensuring adequate coverage during peak periods while avoiding unnecessary overstaffing during quieter times. This predictive approach transforms reactive hospital management into proactive, data-driven operations that improve both efficiency and patient care quality.

Real-time monitoring systems provide continuous oversight of hospital bed availability, enabling dynamic resource management. AI-powered monitoring platforms track bed status across all departments, automatically updating availability as patients are admitted, transferred, or discharged. This eliminates manual tracking errors and provides instant visibility into hospital capacity. Optimized bed allocation algorithms ensure patients receive appropriate placements quickly, reducing wait times in emergency departments and improving patient flow throughout the facility. The system considers factors like patient acuity, required equipment, and staff expertise when making allocation decisions. Real-time bed tracking minimizes delays by immediately identifying available resources and coordinating transfers efficiently. This enhanced visibility improves overall patient care by reducing bottlenecks and ensuring timely access to appropriate accommodations. Hospital staff can make informed decisions quickly, leading to better resource utilization and improved patient satisfaction through reduced waiting periods and more efficient care delivery.

AI-driven bed management directly addresses two critical hospital challenges: excessive wait times and overcrowding. Optimized bed management systems enable efficient allocation by continuously monitoring capacity and predicting future needs, ensuring timely availability when patients require admission. This proactive approach significantly reduces delays that often occur when beds aren't available immediately. Patient influx prediction capabilities allow hospitals to anticipate busy periods and prepare additional resources accordingly, preventing overcrowding situations before they develop. The system analyzes patterns like seasonal variations, local events, and historical data to forecast patient volumes accurately. Improved patient experience results from reduced wait times and less crowded environments, enhancing both patient safety and satisfaction. Shorter wait times decrease patient stress and anxiety while reducing the risk of complications that can occur during extended delays. Less crowded facilities provide better infection control and allow staff to deliver more personalized attention to each patient.

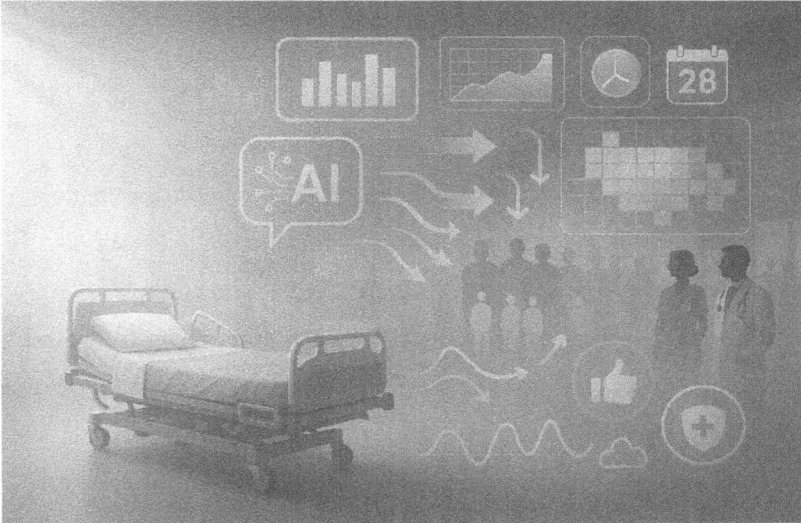

AI-driven staff scheduling revolutionizes workforce management through intelligent analysis and optimization. Shift pattern analysis involves examining historical scheduling data to identify optimal work arrangements that balance hospital operational needs with staff preferences and well-being. The system considers factors like patient acuity patterns, seasonal variations, and staff expertise when creating schedules. Staff availability integration ensures schedules respect personal preferences, time-off requests, and individual constraints while maintaining adequate coverage. This personalized approach improves job satisfaction and reduces scheduling conflicts. Patient volume consideration uses predictive analytics to adapt staffing levels dynamically, ensuring appropriate coverage during peak periods while avoiding overstaffing during slower times. The system can automatically adjust schedules based on predicted patient volumes, emergency situations, or unexpected changes in demand. This intelligent scheduling approach optimizes labor costs while maintaining quality care standards and improving staff satisfaction through more predictable and fair scheduling practices.

Automated task allocation streamlines hospital workflows through intelligent assignment and coordination systems. AI task automation reduces manual intervention by automatically distributing work assignments based on staff availability, expertise, and current workload. This eliminates the time-consuming process of manual task delegation and ensures optimal resource utilization. The system considers factors like staff certifications, current assignments, and location when making allocation decisions. Workflow optimization ensures tasks are completed efficiently by identifying bottlenecks and prioritizing critical activities. The system can automatically sequence tasks to minimize delays and maximize productivity. Error reduction through automated coordination significantly enhances overall task accuracy and reliability by eliminating human oversight mistakes and ensuring consistent processes. Automated systems maintain detailed logs of all activities, enabling quality assurance and continuous improvement. This comprehensive automation approach reduces administrative burden on staff while improving operational efficiency and reducing the likelihood of missed or delayed tasks that could impact patient care.

AI-powered optimization delivers measurable improvements in staff satisfaction and operational cost reduction. Workload optimization algorithms analyze task distribution patterns to balance assignments effectively, reducing employee stress and preventing burnout. The system ensures no individual staff member becomes overwhelmed while maintaining productivity standards. This balanced approach improves job satisfaction by creating more manageable workloads and reducing the pressure that often leads to staff turnover. Scheduling conflict minimization through intelligent algorithms ensures smoother operations and better staff coordination by automatically resolving potential conflicts before they occur. The system considers all constraints and preferences to create harmonious schedules. Operational cost savings result from improved efficiency through optimized resource utilization, reduced overtime expenses, and decreased turnover costs. AI systems eliminate waste in staffing by ensuring appropriate coverage without overstaffing. The combination of happier, less stressed employees and more efficient operations creates a positive cycle that benefits both staff well-being and hospital financial performance.

AI-based forecasting transforms medical supply and pharmaceutical management through sophisticated predictive capabilities. Machine learning algorithms analyze multiple data sources including historical usage patterns, seasonal trends, patient volume fluctuations, and external factors like disease outbreaks or supply chain disruptions. This comprehensive analysis enables accurate demand forecasting that accounts for complex variables affecting supply needs. The algorithms continuously learn from new data, improving prediction accuracy over time. Demand prediction capabilities help ensure medical supplies and pharmaceuticals are stocked proactively rather than reactively, preventing critical shortages that could compromise patient care. The system can predict needs weeks or months in advance, allowing adequate time for procurement and delivery. Proactive inventory management minimizes shortages by maintaining optimal stock levels while avoiding excessive overstock that ties up capital and risks expiration. This balanced approach ensures critical medical supplies remain available when needed while optimizing storage costs and reducing waste from expired products.

AI-driven inventory management addresses the critical balance between preventing shortages and avoiding costly overstock situations. Advanced algorithms analyze consumption patterns, supplier reliability, and demand variability to optimize inventory levels continuously. The system maintains just enough stock to meet projected needs while minimizing carrying costs and storage requirements. Preventing overstock situations avoids costly inventory buildup that ties up valuable capital and increases the risk of product expiration, particularly important for pharmaceuticals with limited shelf lives. Excess inventory also requires additional storage space and management resources. Avoiding supply shortages ensures critical supplies remain available for patient care, preventing delays in treatment or compromised care quality. The system provides early warning alerts when stock levels approach predetermined thresholds, enabling timely reordering. This intelligent approach reduces both the financial risks of excess inventory and the clinical risks of supply shortages, creating optimal inventory management that supports both financial health and patient care quality.

AI optimization extends beyond inventory management to encompass comprehensive procurement and distribution coordination. AI-driven procurement scheduling systems analyze supply availability, vendor performance, and hospital demand patterns to optimize ordering schedules. The system considers factors like lead times, minimum order quantities, and volume discounts to create cost-effective procurement strategies. This intelligent scheduling ensures supplies arrive when needed while minimizing procurement costs through strategic timing and vendor selection. Distribution logistics coordination uses AI to ensure timely delivery of medical supplies throughout the hospital system. The system optimizes delivery routes, schedules, and resource allocation to minimize delays and ensure uninterrupted operations. This includes coordinating internal distribution from central stores to individual departments and managing external deliveries from suppliers. The integrated approach to procurement and distribution creates seamless supply chain operations that support continuous patient care while optimizing costs and minimizing waste through efficient coordination of all supply chain activities.

AI revolutionizes insurance claims processing by automating complex administrative tasks and significantly reducing errors. Claims submission automation streamlines the entire process by automatically extracting relevant information from medical records, populating claim forms accurately, and submitting them to appropriate insurance providers. This eliminates manual data entry errors and accelerates processing times substantially. The system can handle multiple insurance formats and requirements simultaneously. Error reduction through automation significantly improves accuracy and reliability by eliminating human mistakes in claims validation, coding, and submission. AI systems cross-reference medical procedures with appropriate billing codes and verify claim completeness before submission. Faster reimbursements result from accelerated claims validation, reducing the time between service delivery and payment receipt. This improved cash flow benefits both hospitals and patients through quicker resolution of financial obligations. The automation also provides detailed tracking and reporting capabilities, enabling better financial management and reducing the administrative burden on hospital staff.

Machine learning algorithms provide sophisticated fraud detection capabilities that protect hospitals from significant financial losses. These systems analyze billing patterns, claim frequencies, and provider behaviors to identify unusual activities that may indicate fraudulent practices. The algorithms can detect subtle patterns that human reviewers might miss, including irregular billing sequences, unusual procedure combinations, or anomalous claim volumes. Machine learning models continuously adapt to new fraud schemes, improving detection accuracy over time. Early detection of fraudulent activities enables hospitals to address issues before they result in substantial financial damage or regulatory penalties. The system flags suspicious activities for human review while automatically processing clearly legitimate claims. This approach protects hospitals financially by preventing payment of fraudulent claims while maintaining efficient processing of valid reimbursement requests. The fraud detection capabilities also help hospitals maintain compliance with regulatory requirements and avoid penalties associated with fraudulent billing practices, protecting both financial resources and institutional reputation.

AI significantly improves billing accuracy and streamlines revenue cycle management processes. Billing accuracy improvement systems automatically identify and correct common billing discrepancies before claims submission, reducing errors that could delay payment or result in claim rejections. The system validates medical codes, verifies procedure documentation, and ensures compliance with insurance requirements. This proactive approach reduces the costly cycle of claim rejections, corrections, and resubmissions. Optimized revenue cycle management streamlines the entire process from patient registration through final payment collection. AI systems coordinate patient eligibility verification, prior authorization requests, claims submission, and payment posting. This comprehensive approach enhances cash flow by reducing delays at each stage of the revenue cycle. The system provides real-time visibility into revenue cycle performance, identifying bottlenecks and opportunities for improvement. Enhanced financial health results from faster payment collection, reduced administrative costs, and improved cash flow predictability. This optimization enables hospitals to focus resources on patient care rather than administrative complexities while maintaining strong financial performance.

AI transformation of hospital operations delivers comprehensive benefits across all major operational areas. Optimizing hospital operations through AI creates integrated systems that streamline resource management, staffing, supply chains, and billing processes. This holistic approach ensures all hospital functions work together efficiently rather than operating in isolation. The synergy between optimized systems multiplies the benefits achieved in individual areas. Improved efficiency and cost reduction represent immediate tangible benefits of AI implementation. Automated processes reduce manual labor requirements, minimize errors, and accelerate routine tasks. Cost savings result from optimized resource utilization, reduced waste, and improved productivity. These financial benefits provide resources for additional improvements and enhanced patient services. Enhanced patient care outcomes represent the ultimate goal of AI implementation in healthcare. Optimized processes and data-driven decision making directly contribute to better patient experiences, improved safety, reduced wait times, and more personalized care. AI enables hospitals to provide higher quality care while operating more efficiently, creating sustainable improvements that benefit patients, staff, and the broader healthcare system.

Chapter 7: Virtual Health Assistants

Virtual health assistants represent a fundamental shift in healthcare delivery, leveraging artificial intelligence to provide continuous patient support. These systems offer four core functions that address critical healthcare challenges. AI-driven patient support ensures accurate health information is available 24/7, eliminating barriers to basic healthcare guidance. Symptom assessment capabilities help patients understand when professional medical attention is necessary versus when self-care might suffice. Medication reminder systems tackle the significant problem of treatment non-adherence, which affects millions of patients worldwide. Finally, personalized patient guidance creates tailored healthcare experiences that improve engagement and outcomes while supporting care coordination between patients and healthcare providers.

The technological foundation of virtual health assistants relies on four key innovations that enable sophisticated healthcare interactions. Natural Language Processing allows these systems to understand complex patient queries and respond in conversational, accessible language. Machine learning capabilities enable continuous improvement, allowing assistants to learn from interactions and provide increasingly accurate responses over time. Voice recognition technology creates hands-free interaction opportunities, particularly valuable for patients with mobility limitations or during multitasking scenarios. Electronic Health Record integration ensures assistants can access relevant patient data to provide personalized, contextually appropriate guidance while maintaining continuity with existing healthcare systems and provider workflows.

Automated symptom assessment represents a critical first line of healthcare support, utilizing sophisticated algorithms to evaluate patient-reported symptoms. These systems analyze symptom patterns, severity indicators, and associated factors to provide preliminary health assessments that guide patients toward appropriate next steps. Algorithm-based evaluation processes complex symptom combinations more consistently than patients might self-assess, reducing anxiety while providing structured guidance. Preliminary triage recommendations help patients understand whether they need emergency care, should schedule a routine appointment, or can manage symptoms with self-care measures. This systematic approach reduces unnecessary emergency department visits while ensuring patients with serious conditions receive timely attention.

Conversational interfaces transform the traditionally impersonal nature of healthcare technology into engaging, supportive interactions. Interactive patient communication creates real-time, two-way dialogue that feels natural and responsive to individual patient needs and concerns. These systems provide personalized health support by adapting responses based on patient history, current symptoms, and specific circumstances. The accessibility factor is particularly significant, as patients can access health guidance anytime and anywhere, breaking down traditional barriers related to office hours, geographic location, or transportation challenges. This constant availability is especially valuable for patients managing chronic conditions who need ongoing support and reassurance between scheduled appointments.

While symptom checker tools offer significant benefits, understanding their limitations is crucial for safe implementation. Accuracy limitations arise from incomplete data input, algorithm constraints, and the inherent complexity of medical diagnosis, which requires human clinical judgment. The risk of overreliance represents a significant concern, as patients might delay seeking necessary professional medical care based solely on automated assessments. This could lead to missed diagnoses or delayed treatment of serious conditions. Careful implementation requires clear disclaimers about tool limitations, integration with healthcare provider workflows, and patient education about when professional medical consultation remains essential. Effective systems emphasize that they supplement rather than replace professional medical judgment.

Personalized medication scheduling addresses one of healthcare's most persistent challenges: medication non-adherence, which affects up to 50% of patients with chronic conditions. Virtual assistants create customized medication plans that integrate with patients' daily routines, work schedules, and lifestyle preferences, making adherence more achievable. These systems consider factors like meal timing, work hours, and other medications to optimize scheduling for maximum effectiveness and convenience. Timely reminders use context-aware technology to send notifications at the most appropriate moments, considering the patient's location, activity, and previous response patterns. This personalized approach significantly improves adherence rates, leading to better treatment outcomes and reduced healthcare costs.

Adherence monitoring and reporting create a comprehensive feedback loop that benefits both patients and healthcare providers. Advanced tracking systems monitor medication-taking behavior through various methods, including smart pill dispensers, mobile app confirmations, and patient-reported data. These tools identify patterns of non-adherence early, allowing for timely interventions before treatment effectiveness is compromised. Detailed adherence reports provide healthcare providers with objective data about patient compliance, enabling more informed clinical decisions and personalized treatment adjustments. Early intervention capabilities allow providers to address barriers to adherence promptly, whether they're related to side effects, cost concerns, or lifestyle factors, ultimately preventing complications and improving patient outcomes.

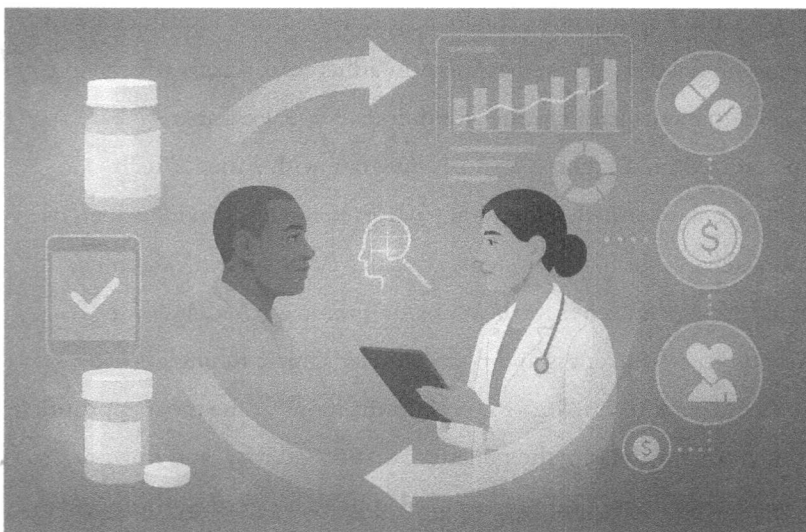

Chapter 7: Virtual Health Assistants

The impact of medication adherence tools extends far beyond simple reminder systems, creating measurable improvements in chronic disease management. Enhanced medication adherence leads to better disease control, as consistent medication intake allows treatments to work as intended by healthcare providers. This improved control directly translates to reduced hospitalizations, as patients with well-managed chronic conditions experience fewer acute exacerbations requiring emergency care. The reduction in hospital visits not only decreases healthcare costs but also reduces strain on healthcare systems, freeing resources for other patient needs. Most importantly, better disease management significantly enhances patients' quality of life, enabling them to maintain independence, continue working, and engage in meaningful activities with greater confidence and fewer health-related limitations.

AI-driven decision support systems represent the next evolution in healthcare triage, processing vast amounts of complex patient data to make accurate care level assessments. These systems analyze multiple data points simultaneously, including symptom severity, patient history, vital signs, and risk factors, to provide comprehensive evaluations that might take human reviewers significantly longer to complete. AI analysis identifies subtle patterns and correlations that could be missed during busy clinical periods. Care level recommendations ensure patients receive appropriate treatment intensity, from self-care guidance to urgent specialist referrals. Optimized resource allocation helps healthcare systems direct their limited resources toward patients with the greatest need, improving overall system efficiency while maintaining high-quality care standards for all patients.

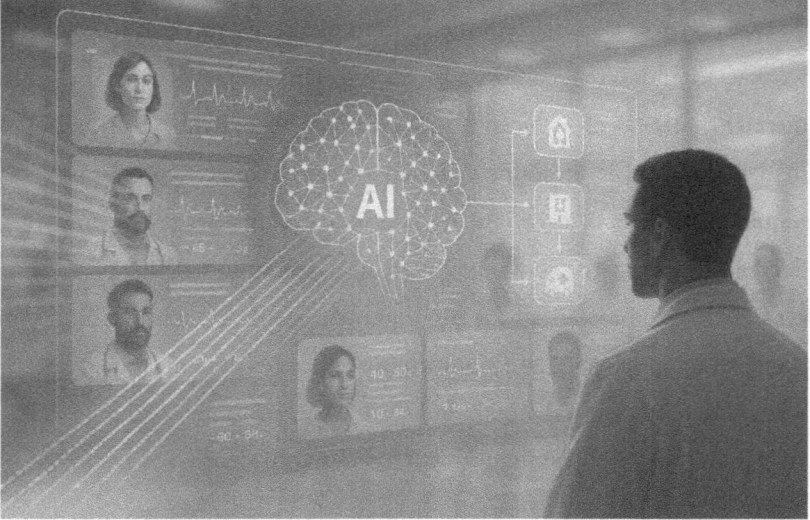

Integration with clinical workflows and EHR systems ensures that AI-powered triage tools enhance rather than disrupt existing healthcare operations. Seamless data integration allows triage information to flow directly into provider systems, eliminating duplicate data entry and reducing the risk of information loss or transcription errors. Enhanced accessibility means clinicians can access AI-generated triage insights within their familiar workflow systems, reducing learning curves and improving adoption rates. This integration supports coordinated care by ensuring all healthcare team members have access to the same triage information, enabling consistent treatment approaches across different departments and care settings. The result is improved care continuity and reduced communication gaps that could compromise patient safety.

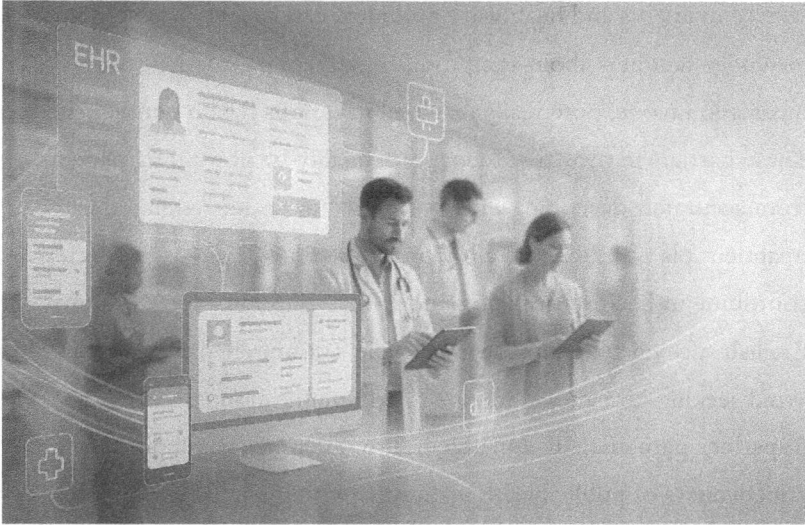

AI-powered triage systems significantly enhance healthcare efficiency while reducing clinician burden in several key ways. Automation of routine assessments frees healthcare professionals from time-consuming preliminary evaluations, allowing them to focus on complex clinical decision-making and direct patient care. This reduction in clinician workload is particularly valuable during high-demand periods, helping prevent burnout while maintaining care quality. By handling initial triage processes, AI systems enable healthcare providers to prioritize their attention toward cases requiring human expertise and empathy. The improved efficiency benefits both clinicians and patients, as reduced wait times and more focused provider attention lead to better healthcare experiences and outcomes for all involved parties.

Language barriers in healthcare create significant challenges that can compromise patient safety and care quality. Communication obstacles between patients and healthcare providers can lead to misunderstandings about symptoms, treatment instructions, or medication usage, potentially resulting in serious health consequences. These barriers particularly impact care quality by preventing patients from accurately describing their symptoms or understanding their treatment plans, leading to suboptimal outcomes. Language differences contribute to health disparities among diverse populations, as non-English speaking patients may receive less comprehensive care or avoid seeking care altogether due to communication concerns. These disparities perpetuate inequitable health outcomes and limit the effectiveness of public health initiatives in multilingual communities.

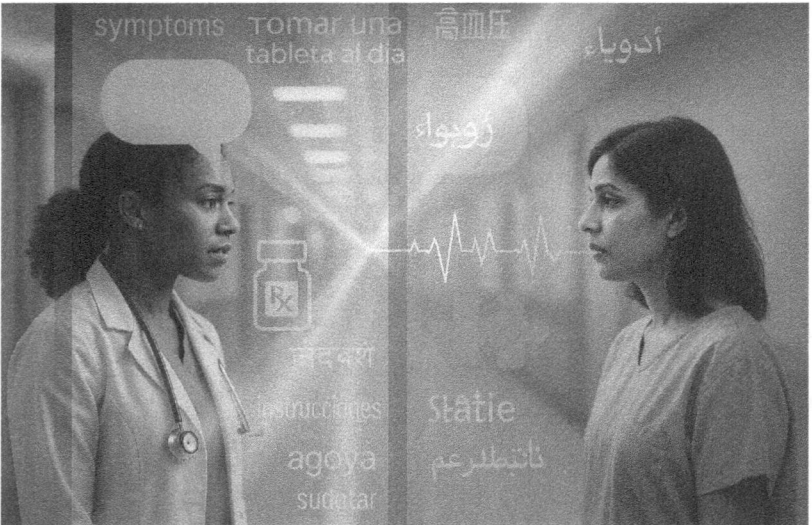

Machine translation and natural language processing technologies offer powerful solutions to overcome language barriers in healthcare settings. Multilingual communication capabilities enable virtual assistants to understand patient queries and provide responses in multiple languages seamlessly, eliminating the need for human interpreters in many routine interactions. Advanced natural language processing improves the clarity and accuracy of translated medical information, ensuring patients receive precise guidance about their health concerns. These technologies facilitate enhanced user support through natural, culturally appropriate conversations that respect linguistic nuances and medical terminology across different languages. The result is more effective healthcare communication that maintains accuracy while providing accessible, understandable guidance to patients regardless of their primary language.

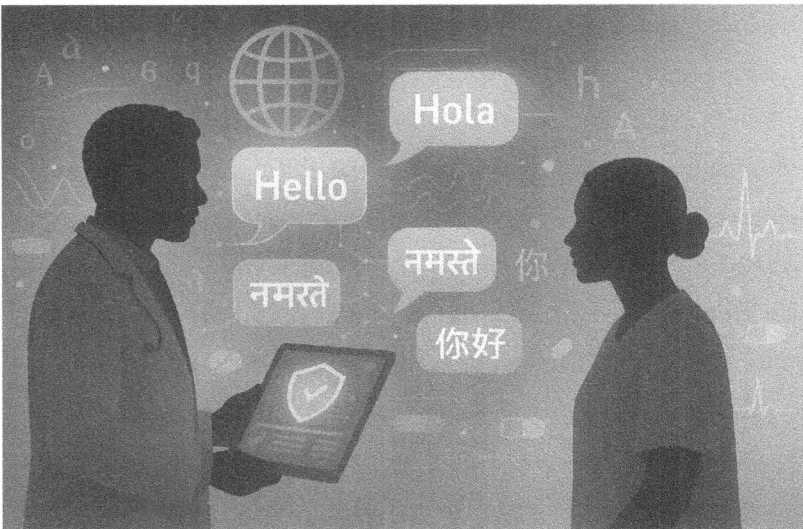

Multilingual virtual health assistants play a crucial role in improving health equity and access for diverse populations. Multilingual support importance cannot be overstated, as it promotes inclusivity by ensuring all patients can access healthcare information and guidance in their preferred language, leading to better understanding and engagement with their care. This technology directly enhances health equity by bridging language gaps that have historically created barriers to quality healthcare access. When patients can communicate effectively with healthcare systems in their native language, disparities in care quality and outcomes are significantly reduced. This improved access leads to better preventive care utilization, earlier intervention for health problems, and more effective chronic disease management across all population groups.

Virtual health assistants represent a transformative force in modern healthcare, delivering benefits across three critical dimensions. Enhanced patient engagement occurs through timely, personalized medical support that meets patients where they are, when they need assistance. These systems provide 24/7 availability and tailored guidance that improves patient satisfaction and treatment adherence. Improved healthcare efficiency results from streamlined workflows, reduced administrative burden on providers, and optimized resource allocation that reduces wait times and improves service delivery. Most importantly, these technologies contribute to better health outcomes by enhancing access to care, supporting medication adherence, facilitating early intervention, and providing personalized guidance that empowers patients to take active roles in managing their health effectively.

Chapter 8: AI in Clinical Research and Trials

AI is currently being applied across three primary domains in clinical research. First, AI for data analysis enables advanced statistical methods and pattern recognition, helping researchers uncover insights that traditional methods might miss. Second, patient monitoring uses AI to continuously track participants' health metrics, improving safety protocols and enabling personalized care adjustments during trials. Third, trial optimization employs machine learning to automate routine administrative tasks, optimize study protocols, and enhance overall trial design efficiency. These applications collectively streamline the research process while maintaining scientific rigor.

The integration of AI in clinical research faces several critical challenges that must be addressed for successful implementation. Data quality challenges are paramount, as AI systems require high-quality, consistent datasets to function effectively, but clinical data often contains inconsistencies and errors. AI interpretability remains crucial for building trust among researchers and regulators who need to understand how algorithms make decisions. Seamless workflow integration is necessary to enhance efficiency without disrupting established clinical processes. However, successfully overcoming these challenges creates significant opportunities for improved research outcomes and innovative healthcare solutions.

Regulatory considerations for AI in clinical research are rapidly evolving as agencies adapt to new technologies. Regulatory frameworks are continuously being updated by organizations like the

FDA and EMA to effectively manage AI applications in clinical trials. Validation and transparency requirements ensure that AI algorithms are rigorously tested and their decision-making processes are explainable to stakeholders. Patient privacy protection remains a top priority, requiring robust data security measures and compliance protocols. Adherence to established guidelines from regulatory agencies ensures legal and ethical use of AI technologies while maintaining public trust in clinical research.

AI-driven trial protocol development represents a significant advancement in clinical research efficiency. Optimized protocol design uses AI to analyze large historical datasets and identify the most effective trial parameters, maximizing both effectiveness and operational efficiency. AI's predictive capabilities help reduce trial duration by forecasting potential outcomes and identifying optimal endpoints earlier in the process. Risk prediction algorithms analyze patient populations and study designs to anticipate potential safety issues or trial complications before they occur. This proactive approach enables researchers to make informed decisions that improve both participant safety and study success rates.

AI significantly enhances patient recruitment and eligibility identification, addressing one of clinical research's biggest bottlenecks. Machine learning algorithms can analyze electronic health records and patient databases to accurately identify individuals who meet specific trial criteria, dramatically improving the precision of patient selection. This enhanced identification capability directly translates to improved recruitment efficiency, reducing the time needed to enroll sufficient participants and accelerating trial initiation. By streamlining eligibility screening processes, AI minimizes trial delays that traditionally plague clinical research, ensuring studies can proceed on schedule and within budget while maintaining appropriate participant selection standards.

AI plays a crucial role in improving diversity and representation in clinical trials, addressing historical inequities in medical research. AI identification tools analyze demographic and clinical data to identify patient groups that have been underrepresented in previous studies, ensuring more inclusive recruitment strategies. These insights enable researchers to develop targeted approaches for enhancing trial diversity, implementing strategies that actively recruit from varied populations across different demographics, geographic regions, and socioeconomic backgrounds. Greater diversity in clinical trials leads to more generalizable results that better represent the broader population, ultimately improving the applicability and effectiveness of medical treatments across all patient groups.

Natural Language Processing revolutionizes clinical data extraction from medical publications, automating what has traditionally been a time-intensive manual process. NLP algorithms can efficiently process vast amounts of medical literature, automatically extracting relevant clinical data points, study results, and key findings from published research. This automation significantly improves both efficiency and accuracy by reducing time consumption and minimizing human errors that commonly occur during manual data extraction processes. The technology enables researchers to quickly synthesize information from hundreds or thousands of publications, accelerating evidence-based decision making and reducing the risk of overlooking important research findings.

Chapter 8: AI in Clinical Research and Trials

AI-powered summarization tools efficiently condense large volumes of research literature into clear, concise summaries that researchers can quickly digest. These intelligent systems can process extensive databases of medical publications, identifying key themes, methodologies, and findings across multiple studies. The resulting summaries provide significant benefits to researchers by helping them stay informed about the latest evidence and scientific developments in their fields without requiring exhaustive manual literature reviews. This capability is particularly valuable in rapidly evolving medical fields where staying current with new research is essential for informed decision-making and study design.

Natural Language Processing enhances systematic reviews and meta-analyses by automating critical components of the research synthesis process. Efficient study identification uses NLP algorithms to automatically search and identify relevant studies from vast literature databases, saving considerable time and reducing manual effort. Improved screening accuracy is achieved through sophisticated content analysis that categorizes and selects studies based on predetermined criteria with greater consistency than human reviewers. Faster data synthesis enables NLP to accelerate the combination and analysis of data from multiple studies, enhancing both the quality and speed of meta-analyses while maintaining rigorous methodological standards.

Leveraging electronic health record data through AI processing unlocks valuable insights about patient treatments and real-world outcomes. AI data analysis capabilities can process massive volumes of EHR data to identify patterns and correlations that inform evidence-based medical decisions. Treatment effectiveness assessment becomes more comprehensive as insights from real-world data complement traditional clinical trial results, providing a broader understanding of how interventions perform in diverse patient populations. Patient safety and outcomes analysis using health records enables researchers to identify potential adverse events, monitor treatment responses, and continuously improve healthcare delivery based on actual patient experiences rather than controlled trial conditions alone.

Predictive analytics represents a powerful application of machine learning in healthcare, enabling personalized treatment approaches based on individual patient characteristics. Machine learning models analyze comprehensive patient data including demographics, medical history, genetic information, and real-time health metrics to predict treatment responses and identify potential health risks. These predictive insights directly support personalized treatment decisions by helping clinicians select optimal interventions for individual patients based on their unique risk profiles and predicted outcomes. The implementation of predictive models leads to improved clinical outcomes through proactive risk assessment and tailored treatment strategies that address individual patient needs more effectively.

Continuous learning systems for post-market surveillance represent the next evolution in drug and device safety monitoring. AI-driven monitoring systems continuously analyze post-market data streams including adverse event reports, electronic health records, and real-world usage patterns to detect safety signals and adverse events as they emerge. Real-time safety updates enable these systems to instantly update safety profiles and risk assessments as new data becomes available, providing healthcare providers and regulators with current information about emerging risks. This continuous monitoring approach significantly improves patient safety by identifying potential issues much earlier than traditional surveillance methods, enabling rapid response to emerging safety concerns.

Synthetic control arms utilize historical or real-world data to create comparator groups in clinical trials, representing a paradigm shift in trial design. This approach reduces or eliminates the need for traditional placebo control groups by leveraging existing data to establish baseline comparisons for experimental interventions. The reduction of placebo controls addresses ethical concerns about withholding potentially beneficial treatments from patients while maintaining scientific rigor. Synthetic control arms significantly increase trial efficiency by accelerating data collection processes and reducing operational costs associated with recruiting and maintaining large control populations, while still providing robust statistical comparisons for regulatory approval.

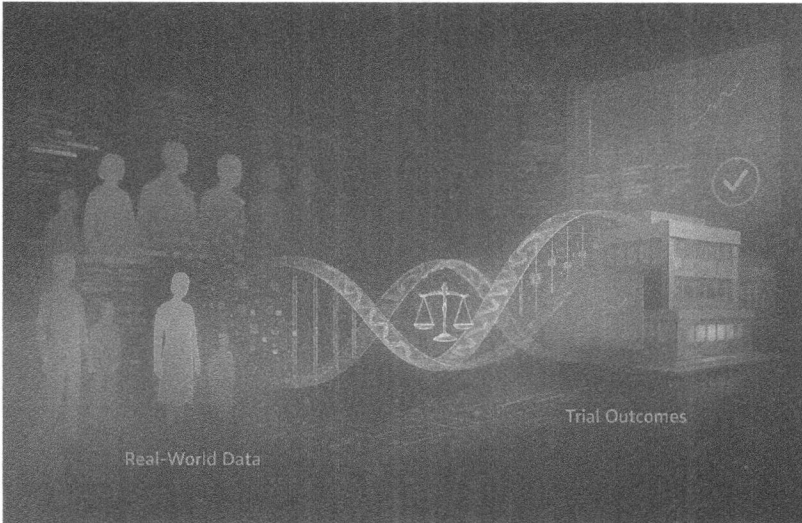

AI-driven creation of simulated patient cohorts represents an innovative approach to addressing recruitment challenges in clinical research. These systems generate realistic patient cohorts that closely resemble actual trial populations in terms of demographics, medical history, and relevant characteristics, ensuring study accuracy and validity. Simulated cohorts provide robust support for hypothesis testing by offering consistent and controlled trial populations that can be used to validate study designs and statistical approaches before implementing full-scale trials. This approach significantly reduces recruitment challenges by supplementing or, in some cases, substituting for traditional patient enrollment, particularly valuable for rare disease studies where patient populations are limited.

Ethical and regulatory considerations for simulated trials require careful attention to maintain research integrity and public trust. Data integrity concerns focus on ensuring the accuracy and trustworthiness of simulated trial data, requiring rigorous validation methods to demonstrate that synthetic data accurately represents real-world patient populations and treatment responses. Patient consent issues remain complex even in simulated environments, as researchers must address questions about using historical patient data and obtaining appropriate permissions. Regulatory acceptance requires meeting rigorous standards and guidelines established by agencies like the FDA and EMA, who must evaluate the validity and reliability of simulated trial outcomes before approving new treatments based on synthetic evidence.

AI's transformative potential in clinical research extends across all phases of medical research, from initial study design through post-market surveillance. Artificial intelligence enhances clinical trial design by optimizing protocols and improving patient matching, revolutionizes data analysis through advanced analytics and pattern recognition, and accelerates evidence generation through automated literature reviews and real-world data analysis. The successful integration of AI within established ethical and regulatory frameworks ensures that these technological advances maintain the highest standards of patient safety, data integrity, and scientific rigor. This balanced approach enables innovative clinical research practices that advance medical knowledge while preserving public trust and regulatory compliance.

Chapter 9: Regulatory and Ethical Considerations

Regulatory frameworks for healthcare AI establish three fundamental pillars for safe implementation. Safety and efficacy standards ensure that AI systems undergo rigorous testing and validation before deployment, protecting patients from potentially harmful technologies. Patient protection measures emphasize privacy safeguards, data security protocols, and ethical guidelines that respect individual rights. Compliance and integration requirements provide clear pathways for healthcare organizations to adopt AI tools responsibly. Understanding these frameworks is essential for developers, clinicians, and administrators who must navigate complex regulatory landscapes while maintaining focus on patient welfare and clinical effectiveness.

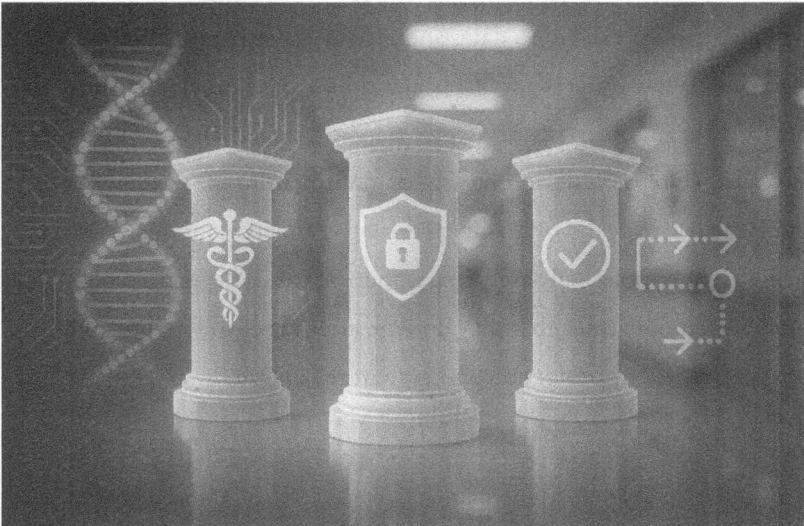

Ethical principles serve as the foundation for responsible AI development and deployment in healthcare. Beneficence and nonmaleficence require that AI systems actively promote positive patient outcomes while preventing harm through careful design and testing. Autonomy principles ensure that patients retain decision-making authority regarding AI-enabled treatments, preserving their right to informed choice. Justice and privacy considerations mandate fair access to AI benefits across diverse populations while protecting sensitive health information. These principles work together to create a comprehensive ethical framework that guides AI development teams, healthcare providers, and policy makers in creating systems that serve all patients equitably and safely.

FDA regulatory pathways for healthcare AI involve comprehensive evaluation processes designed to ensure patient safety and clinical effectiveness. Premarket submissions require developers to provide extensive documentation demonstrating their AI systems' safety profiles, clinical validation data, and intended use parameters. This rigorous review process evaluates algorithms, training data quality, and performance metrics across diverse patient populations. Post-market surveillance represents an ongoing commitment to monitoring AI performance in real-world clinical settings. This continuous oversight helps identify potential safety issues, performance degradation, or unexpected outcomes that may emerge after deployment, ensuring long-term patient protection and system reliability.

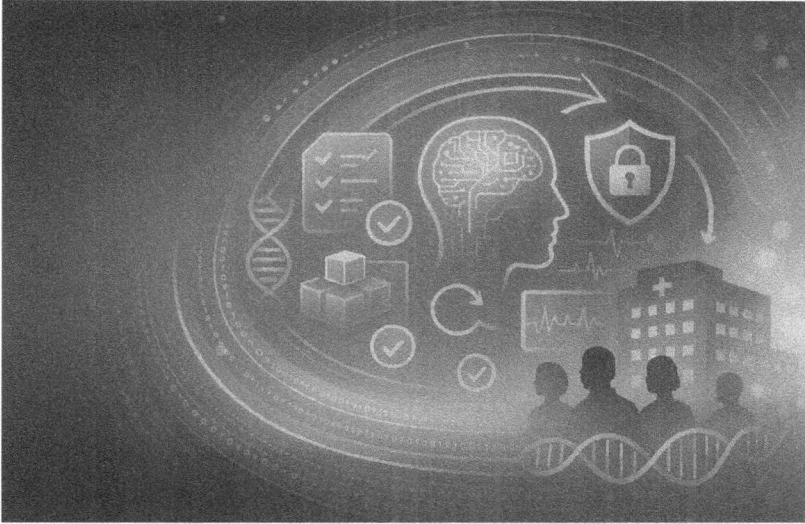

The European Medicines Agency takes a structured approach to AI approval that emphasizes regulatory conformity and risk management. EMA ensures AI technologies comply with existing EU medical device regulations, creating consistency within the broader regulatory framework. Risk assessment receives particular emphasis, with thorough evaluation of potential hazards associated with AI applications before approval. This includes examining algorithmic transparency, data quality, and clinical validation evidence. EMA's process aligns closely with established EU medical device directives, ensuring coherent standards across all medical technologies. This alignment provides clarity for developers while maintaining rigorous safety standards that protect European patients and healthcare systems.

AI tool approval processes face significant challenges that require adaptive regulatory approaches. Algorithm updates and data variability create ongoing complexities, as AI systems may evolve through learning or require modifications based on new evidence. Regulators must balance innovation with safety while developing frameworks for managing these dynamic technologies. Transparency issues present another major challenge, as complex AI algorithms often operate as "black boxes" that are difficult to interpret. Building trust requires clear explanations of AI decision-making processes. Real-world case studies demonstrate successful navigation strategies, showing how collaboration between developers, regulators, and clinicians can overcome these challenges through careful planning, documentation, and ongoing communication.

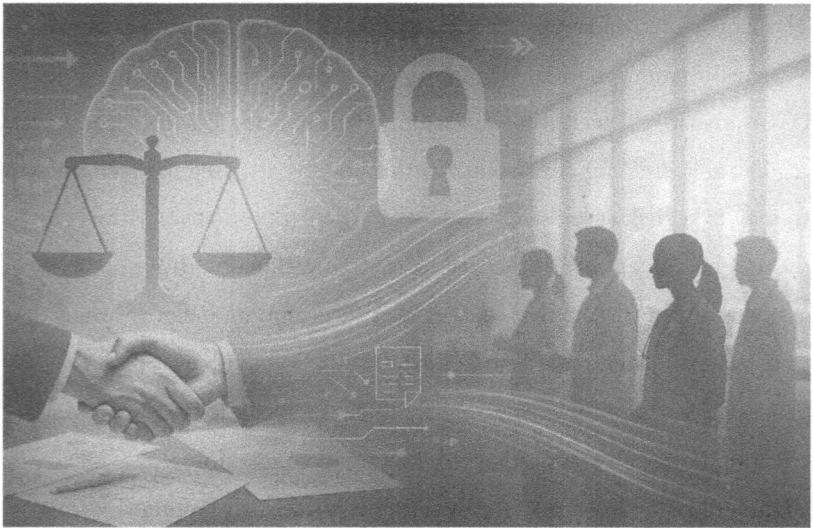

Bias in healthcare AI can emerge from multiple sources, each requiring specific attention and mitigation strategies. Unrepresentative datasets pose significant risks when training data fails to include diverse populations, potentially leading to AI systems that perform poorly for underrepresented groups. This can perpetuate or amplify existing healthcare disparities. Flawed data labeling introduces systematic errors that bias algorithm outputs, affecting diagnostic accuracy and treatment recommendations. Algorithmic design bias occurs when development teams inadvertently incorporate assumptions or limitations that favor certain populations over others. Understanding these bias sources is crucial for developing fair AI systems that serve all patients equitably and provide reliable clinical decision support across diverse healthcare settings.

Effective bias detection and mitigation requires systematic approaches implemented throughout the AI development lifecycle. Data balancing techniques ensure training datasets adequately represent diverse populations, reducing the likelihood of biased outputs. Algorithmic audits provide systematic evaluation methods for detecting bias in AI systems, examining performance across different demographic groups and clinical scenarios. Fairness constraints can be built into AI models during development, establishing rules that promote equitable decision-making. Continuous monitoring tracks model performance over time, identifying emerging bias patterns that may develop as populations or medical practices change. These techniques work together to create comprehensive bias mitigation strategies that support equitable healthcare delivery.

Promoting equity and fairness in AI applications requires proactive strategies that engage diverse stakeholders throughout the development process. Proactive design choices involve considering fairness implications from the earliest stages of AI development, rather than addressing bias as an afterthought. This includes diverse team composition, inclusive design principles, and equity-focused testing protocols. Stakeholder engagement ensures that AI solutions incorporate perspectives from various healthcare communities, including patients, clinicians, and advocacy groups representing underserved populations. Validation across populations involves testing AI systems with diverse demographic groups to identify potential performance disparities. These approaches help prevent discriminatory outcomes and promote AI systems that benefit all patients regardless of background or characteristics.

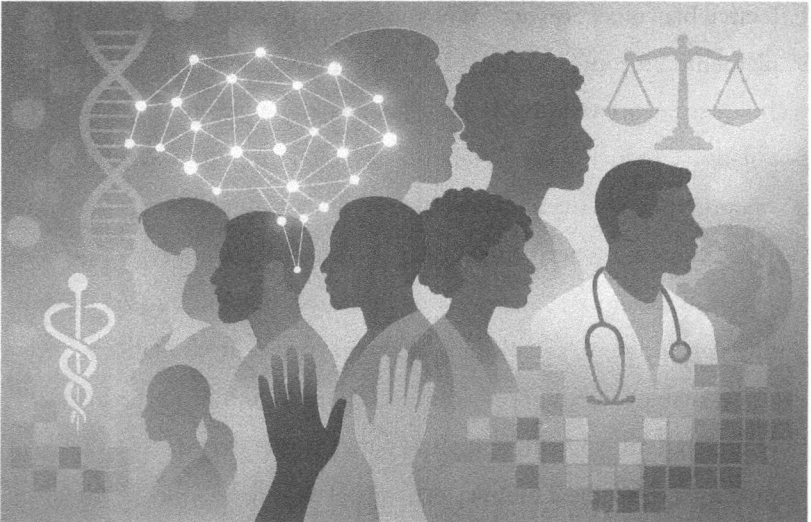

Informed consent in AI-driven clinical decision-making requires clear communication about artificial intelligence's role in patient care. Patient awareness involves explaining how AI systems contribute to diagnosis, treatment recommendations, or care coordination in understandable terms. Healthcare providers must discuss both potential benefits, such as improved diagnostic accuracy or personalized treatment options, and possible risks, including algorithmic errors or limitations. This balanced presentation enables patients to make truly informed decisions about their care. Respecting autonomy means ensuring patients understand their right to decline AI-assisted care when alternatives exist. Effective informed consent processes build trust between patients and providers while upholding ethical principles that respect individual choice and self-determination in healthcare decisions.

Increasing transparency in AI systems requires multiple complementary strategies that make complex technologies more understandable to users. Clear communication involves using straightforward language to explain AI functionality, avoiding technical jargon that may confuse patients or clinicians. Explainable models are designed with interpretability in mind, allowing users to understand how AI systems reach their conclusions. Process documentation provides comprehensive records of AI development, validation, and deployment procedures, supporting transparency and reproducibility. Engagement with users involves ongoing dialogue between AI developers, healthcare providers, and patients to ensure systems meet real-world needs. These strategies work together to create AI systems that are not only technically sound but also trustworthy and accessible to all stakeholders.

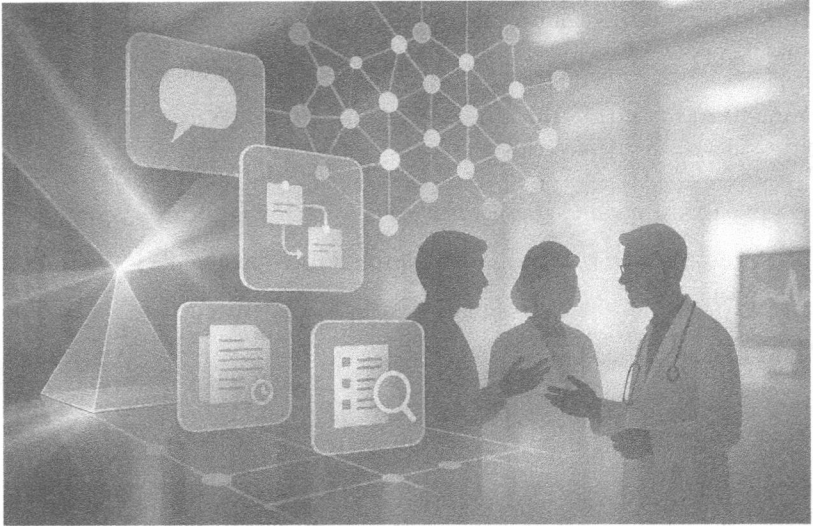

Transparency in patient care creates both opportunities and challenges that require careful consideration of legal and ethical frameworks. Building trust through transparency enhances relationships between healthcare providers and patients by demonstrating openness about AI involvement in care decisions. However, transparency raises important data privacy concerns, as sharing information about AI processes may potentially expose sensitive patient information or proprietary algorithms. Legal and ethical frameworks provide guidance for managing these competing interests, establishing standards for transparency that protect both patient privacy and intellectual property rights. Healthcare organizations must navigate these complex requirements while maintaining transparency levels that support patient trust and informed decision-making without compromising privacy or security obligations.

Chapter 9: Regulatory and Ethical Considerations

Explainability serves critical functions for both clinicians and patients in healthcare AI applications. Clinician understanding enables healthcare providers to comprehend AI recommendations, fostering appropriate trust and effective integration of AI insights into clinical workflow. When clinicians understand how AI systems reach conclusions, they can better evaluate recommendations and make informed decisions about patient care. Patient confidence develops when clear explanations help individuals understand how AI contributes to their care decisions, promoting acceptance and engagement with AI-assisted treatments. Informed decision-making becomes possible when both clinicians and patients have access to comprehensible explanations of AI reasoning. This shared understanding improves healthcare outcomes by ensuring all stakeholders can effectively participate in the care process.

Several methods can enhance AI explainability, each addressing different aspects of interpretability challenges. Model simplification involves designing AI systems with inherently understandable decision processes, though this may require balancing complexity with performance. Visualizations provide powerful tools for illustrating AI reasoning through charts, graphs, and interactive displays that make complex algorithms more accessible. Example-based explanations help users understand AI decisions by showing similar cases and their outcomes, providing concrete context for abstract algorithmic processes. Interpretable models prioritize transparency from the development stage, ensuring that AI reasoning remains comprehensible throughout the system lifecycle. These complementary approaches allow developers to create AI systems that maintain high performance while remaining understandable to healthcare users.

Building and maintaining trust in AI-powered healthcare requires ongoing attention to multiple interconnected factors. Consistent performance establishes confidence through reliable, accurate AI systems that perform predictably across various clinical scenarios and patient populations. Transparency in AI decision-making builds trust by providing clear explanations of how systems reach conclusions, enabling users to understand and verify AI recommendations. Ethical AI practices ensure patient privacy protection and fair treatment across all demographic groups, demonstrating commitment to responsible technology use. Ongoing dialogue among stakeholders promotes mutual understanding and trust through continuous communication between developers, clinicians, patients, and regulatory bodies. These elements work together to create sustainable trust relationships that support successful AI adoption in healthcare settings.

Regulatory approvals ensure that AI systems meet rigorous safety and efficacy standards before deployment, protecting patients through comprehensive evaluation processes. Addressing fairness and obtaining proper informed consent promotes equity in healthcare AI applications, ensuring that all patients benefit from AI technologies while maintaining their autonomy and rights. Transparency and explainability requirements build trust and accountability by making AI systems understandable to both healthcare providers and patients. Success in healthcare AI depends on integrating these considerations throughout the development and deployment lifecycle, creating systems that are not only technically advanced but also safe, fair, and trustworthy for all stakeholders.

Chapter 10: AI Workforce Transformation

AI adoption in healthcare is transforming the industry through four key areas. In diagnostics, machine learning algorithms analyze medical data with unprecedented speed and accuracy, enhancing clinical decision-making. Treatment planning benefits from AI's ability to integrate clinical data with predictive analytics, enabling truly personalized patient care. Administrative automation is reducing manual workloads and improving operational efficiency across healthcare settings. However, adoption varies significantly across institutions and specialties due to differences in technological readiness, financial resources, and clinical needs. This variability creates both opportunities and challenges as organizations at different stages of AI maturity work toward common goals of improved patient outcomes.

The transformation of healthcare workforces is driven primarily by two factors: improving patient outcomes and enhancing operational efficiency. These drivers create compelling business cases for AI investment. However, significant challenges emerge during implementation. Resistance to change remains a major hurdle, as healthcare professionals may fear job displacement or struggle with new technologies. Data privacy concerns are paramount given the sensitive nature of health information and regulatory requirements. Additionally, the need for new skills creates training demands that strain resources and time. Successfully addressing these challenges requires comprehensive change management strategies, robust training programs, and clear communication about AI's role as a tool to augment rather than replace human expertise.

AI integration creates profound implications for healthcare professionals and organizations. Traditional roles and responsibilities are evolving as AI reshapes daily workflows, requiring professionals to manage new tools and incorporate data-driven decision-making into clinical practice. The need for AI competencies has become critical, with healthcare professionals requiring skills in data interpretation, algorithm understanding, and AI output analysis. Organizations must implement comprehensive strategies to support this workforce adaptation while maintaining quality care standards. This includes developing training programs, creating new role definitions, establishing governance frameworks, and fostering cultures that embrace technological innovation. Success requires coordinated efforts across all organizational levels, from executive leadership to frontline staff.

Clinicians require four essential AI-related competencies for effective healthcare integration. Data literacy skills form the foundation, enabling accurate interpretation and application of data in clinical settings. Understanding AI algorithms helps clinicians comprehend how these systems support and influence clinical decisions, building trust and appropriate usage. The ability to skillfully interpret AI outputs is crucial for improving patient outcomes and avoiding misapplication of AI recommendations. Finally, understanding ethical considerations ensures responsible AI integration, protecting patient rights and maintaining professional standards. These competencies work synergistically, creating a comprehensive skill set that enables clinicians to leverage AI effectively while maintaining their critical role in patient care and clinical judgment.

Healthcare organizations can implement AI training through four complementary approaches. Formal education programs, including structured degrees and certificates, provide comprehensive, in-depth knowledge of AI applications in medicine. Online courses and workshops offer flexible, accessible training options that accommodate busy clinical schedules while delivering interactive learning experiences. Hands-on experience with real-world AI tools proves invaluable for building practical skills and integrating AI capabilities with existing clinical expertise. Tailored curricula that combine clinical knowledge with AI fundamentals create the most effective learning outcomes, ensuring relevance to specific healthcare contexts. The most successful programs combine multiple approaches, allowing learners to progress from theoretical understanding to practical application while maintaining clinical focus.

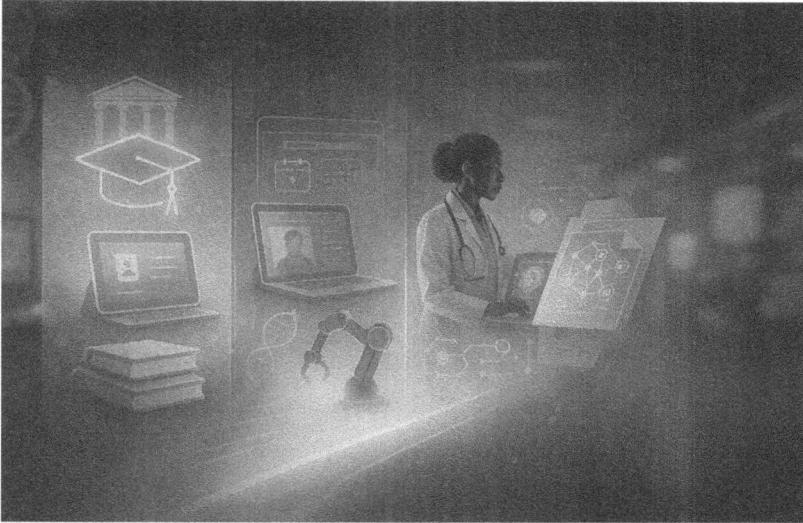

Successful upskilling programs demonstrate three critical elements that drive effective AI adoption. Interdisciplinary training enhances collaboration and knowledge sharing across healthcare fields, breaking down silos and fostering integrated approaches to patient care. Mentorship support plays a pivotal role during AI adoption, providing guidance, encouragement, and practical assistance as clinicians develop new skills and confidence with AI technologies. Continuous learning programs help maintain current skills as AI technologies evolve rapidly, ensuring long-term competency and adaptation. These elements create supportive environments where healthcare professionals can successfully transition to AI-enhanced practice while maintaining high standards of patient care and professional development.

Effective communication serves as the critical bridge between clinical and data science teams, enabling aligned goals, shared expectations, and successful project outcomes. Clear communication channels help translate clinical needs into technical requirements while ensuring data scientists understand healthcare contexts and constraints. Mutual understanding creates shared vocabularies and common frameworks essential for successful AI implementations. When teams develop this mutual understanding, they can navigate complex healthcare challenges more effectively, avoid costly misunderstandings, and create AI solutions that truly serve clinical needs. This communication foundation supports all other collaborative activities and directly impacts project success rates and user adoption of AI technologies.

Interdisciplinary teamwork in AI-driven healthcare projects requires three essential components working in harmony. Clinical expertise provides crucial knowledge for developing AI solutions that are accurate, relevant, and applicable to real healthcare needs and workflows. Data science skills contribute the technical capabilities necessary to design, develop, and optimize AI algorithms specifically for medical applications and healthcare environments. Collaborative development processes ensure that AI tools are both technically sound and clinically usable in real healthcare settings. When these elements combine effectively, teams create AI solutions that seamlessly integrate into clinical practice, improve patient outcomes, and gain acceptance from healthcare professionals who ultimately determine implementation success.

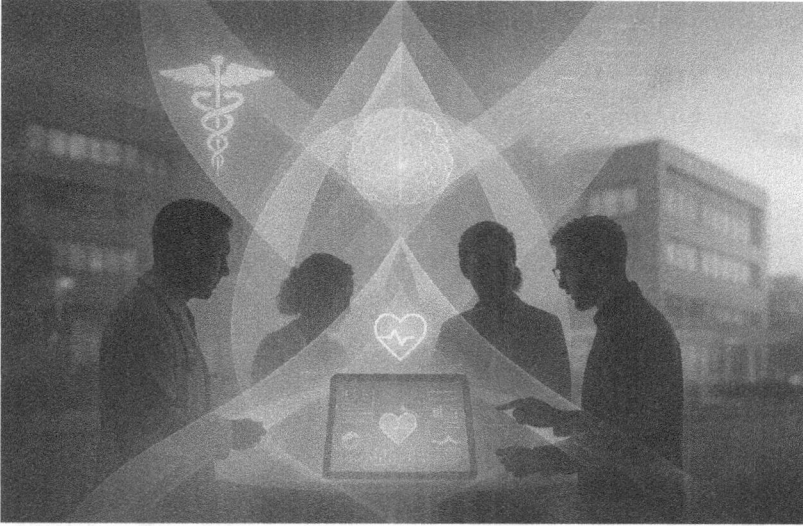

Effective clinician-data scientist collaboration relies on four fundamental best practices. Clear role definition helps team members understand their responsibilities and contributions, reducing confusion and improving coordination throughout project lifecycles. Regular communication ensures ongoing alignment, enables prompt problem identification and resolution, and maintains momentum during complex, long-term projects. Joint problem-solving sessions integrate clinical insights with data expertise, creating more comprehensive and practical solutions than either discipline could develop independently. Fostering mutual trust strengthens teamwork, encourages open communication about challenges and concerns, and ultimately leads to more successful AI project outcomes that serve both technical excellence and clinical needs.

The healthcare industry is witnessing the emergence of three critical new roles that support AI integration. Clinical AI specialists focus specifically on integrating AI tools into healthcare workflows, serving as bridges between technology and clinical practice while improving diagnosis and treatment processes. Data stewards manage and protect healthcare data, ensuring accuracy, compliance with regulations, and appropriate access for AI applications while maintaining patient privacy and security. AI ethicists ensure that AI applications in healthcare are implemented and used ethically and responsibly, protecting patient rights and addressing bias, fairness, and transparency concerns. These roles represent new career paths and essential functions for successful AI adoption.

Traditional healthcare job descriptions require fundamental updates to reflect AI integration realities. Evolving clinical roles now include responsibilities for overseeing and interpreting AI outputs, integrating technology into everyday healthcare practices, and maintaining clinical oversight of AI-assisted decisions. Updated job descriptions must explicitly include AI-related competencies, collaborative responsibilities with technical teams, and data management skills as core requirements rather than optional additions. The emphasis on collaboration and shared responsibility between clinicians and AI technology has become essential for improved patient care, safety, and quality outcomes. Organizations must proactively revise role definitions to attract qualified candidates and set clear performance expectations in AI-enhanced environments.

The future of AI-integrated healthcare environments demands three critical organizational capabilities. Ongoing learning becomes paramount as continuous education enables healthcare workers to keep pace with rapidly evolving AI technologies, ensuring sustained enhancement of patient care capabilities. Flexibility in practice requires adapting workflows, embracing new AI systems, and maintaining effective healthcare delivery in increasingly dynamic technological environments. Proactive change management involves anticipating and systematically managing changes driven by AI advancements, supporting sustained patient-centered care while navigating technological transformation. Organizations that develop these capabilities will thrive in AI-integrated healthcare environments, while those that resist adaptation may struggle to maintain competitiveness and quality standards.

In conclusion, AI transformation in healthcare requires comprehensive attention to three interconnected areas. The transformation of healthcare skills emphasizes adaptability and technology proficiency as essential competencies for all healthcare workers, from entry-level positions to senior leadership roles. AI fosters enhanced collaboration by enabling clinicians to work more efficiently with both technology and each other, creating synergistic relationships that improve patient care quality and outcomes. Upskilling for AI integration through continuous training programs remains critical for successful AI adoption and improved patient outcomes. Organizations that invest in comprehensive workforce development, foster collaborative cultures, and maintain commitment to ongoing learning will successfully navigate this transformation and emerge as leaders in AI-enhanced healthcare delivery.

Chapter 11: Future Trends and Innovations

Our first major topic focuses on generative AI in clinical decision support. This represents one of the most promising applications of artificial intelligence in healthcare, where machine learning models can generate insights, recommendations, and treatment strategies based on vast amounts of medical data. We'll explore how these systems enhance diagnostic accuracy, personalize treatment plans, and address the critical challenges of implementation in clinical settings.

Generative AI is transforming diagnostic accuracy through sophisticated data-driven recommendations. These advanced AI systems process enormous medical datasets to identify subtle patterns that might escape human observation, significantly enhancing diagnostic precision. By serving as intelligent clinical assistants, these systems suggest possible diagnoses based on comprehensive analysis of patient information and existing medical literature. The result is a substantial reduction in diagnostic errors, which historically affect millions of patients annually, leading to improved patient outcomes and more confident clinical decision-making across healthcare settings.

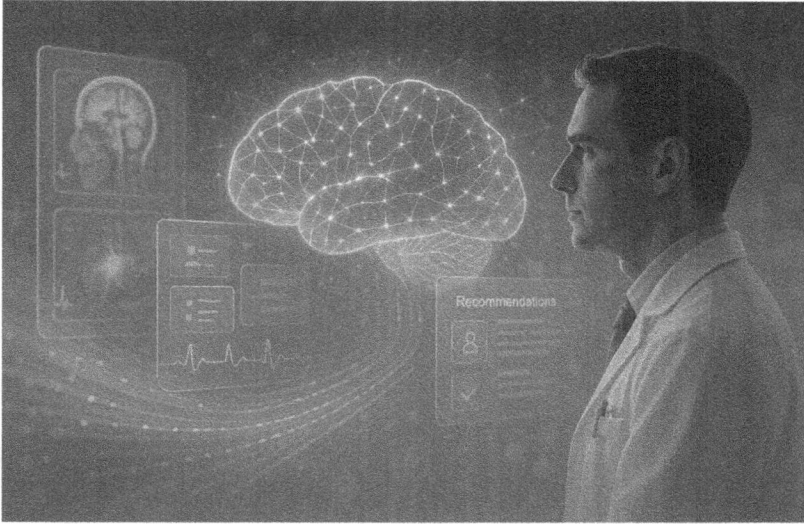

Personalized medicine reaches new heights through generative algorithms that create highly customized treatment plans. These AI systems analyze each patient's unique health profile, including medical history, current symptoms, lifestyle factors, and importantly, genetic information. By incorporating genetics-based healthcare approaches, AI can significantly improve treatment precision and effectiveness, moving beyond one-size-fits-all approaches. This personalization leads to more targeted interventions, reduced adverse effects, and substantially better health outcomes for patients, representing a fundamental shift toward truly individualized medical care.

Despite tremendous potential, generative AI implementation faces significant challenges and ethical considerations that must be carefully addressed. Patient privacy concerns remain paramount, as these systems must protect sensitive medical information while maintaining trust and complying with strict healthcare regulations like HIPAA.

Algorithmic bias presents another critical issue, where biased training data can lead to unfair treatment recommendations and exacerbate healthcare disparities. Transparency becomes essential for fostering accountability in clinical use, ensuring healthcare providers understand and can explain AI-driven decisions to patients and colleagues.

Our second major focus examines autonomous AI agents in healthcare. These sophisticated systems operate independently to monitor patients, assist with routine care tasks, and make real-time decisions about patient safety. Unlike traditional AI tools that require constant human oversight, autonomous agents can function with minimal supervision while maintaining high safety standards, representing a significant advancement in healthcare technology automation.

Autonomous AI agents are revolutionizing patient monitoring and care through three key applications. Continuous vital monitoring systems provide real-time, round-the-clock surveillance of patient vital signs, ensuring timely detection of any health changes that might require immediate attention. Early anomaly detection capabilities enable these systems to identify potential health issues before they become critical, allowing for prompt medical interventions and significantly improved patient safety. Additionally, these agents assist healthcare providers with routine patient care tasks, enhancing overall efficiency and responsiveness while freeing clinical staff to focus on complex decision-making and patient interaction.

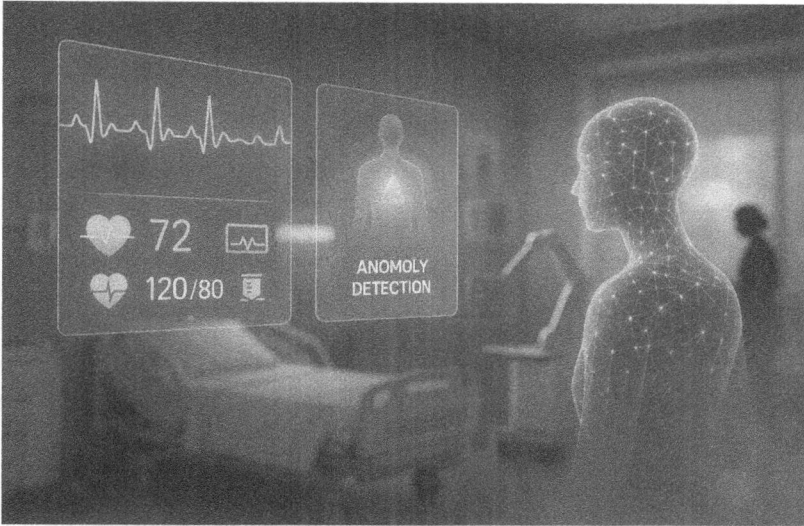

Integration with electronic health records and hospital workflows represents a crucial advancement in healthcare AI implementation. AI agents connect seamlessly with existing EHR systems, dramatically improving accessibility and management of patient data across departments and care teams. This integration enhances clinical decision-making by providing healthcare providers with comprehensive data insights that support timely and accurate treatment decisions. The streamlined hospital workflows resulting from AI automation reduce clinician workload significantly, minimize administrative burdens, and improve operational efficiency throughout healthcare facilities, ultimately leading to better resource utilization and patient care.

Ensuring safety, transparency, and regulatory compliance remains absolutely critical for autonomous AI deployment in healthcare settings. Strict safety protocols must be implemented to guarantee that autonomous AI operates without risking patient health or compromising data integrity. Algorithm transparency builds essential trust by allowing clear understanding of AI decision-making processes, enabling healthcare providers to validate and explain automated recommendations. Regulatory compliance with healthcare standards and regulations protects patients while ensuring legal deployment of AI technology, requiring ongoing collaboration between technology developers, healthcare institutions, and regulatory bodies to maintain the highest safety and ethical standards.

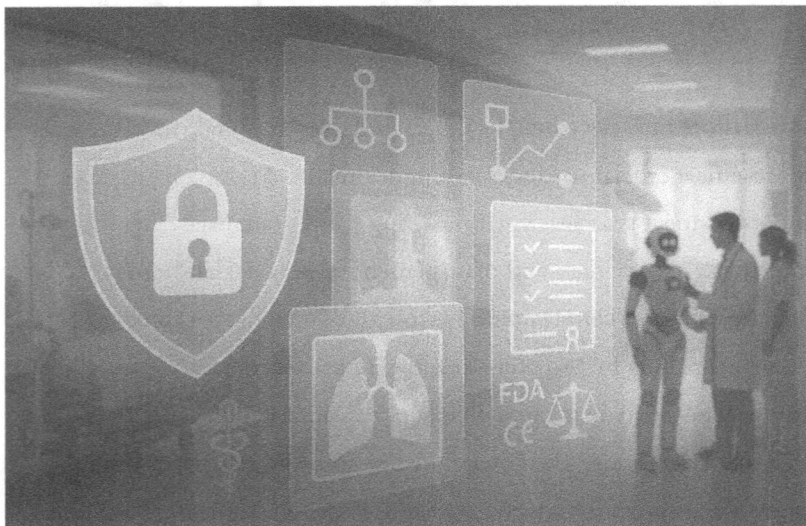

Multimodal AI for integrated diagnosis represents our third major innovation area. This approach combines multiple types of medical data - including imaging, genomics, and clinical information - to create comprehensive diagnostic insights. By processing diverse data sources simultaneously, these systems provide a more complete picture of patient health than any single diagnostic method could achieve alone.

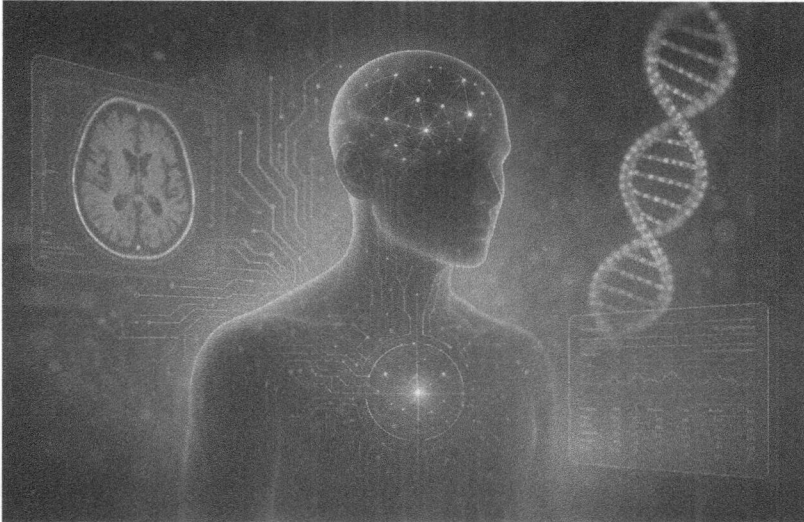

Multimodal data integration revolutionizes healthcare by combining imaging, genomics, and clinical data for comprehensive patient analysis. This holistic approach offers healthcare providers a complete patient view that significantly improves diagnostic accuracy and clinical insights. By integrating multiple biological data layers, these systems enable enhanced diagnostic precision through nuanced diagnoses specifically tailored to individual patient health profiles. Rather than relying on isolated test results or single imaging studies, healthcare providers can now access integrated assessments that consider genetic predispositions, imaging findings, laboratory results, and clinical history simultaneously for more accurate and personalized medical care.

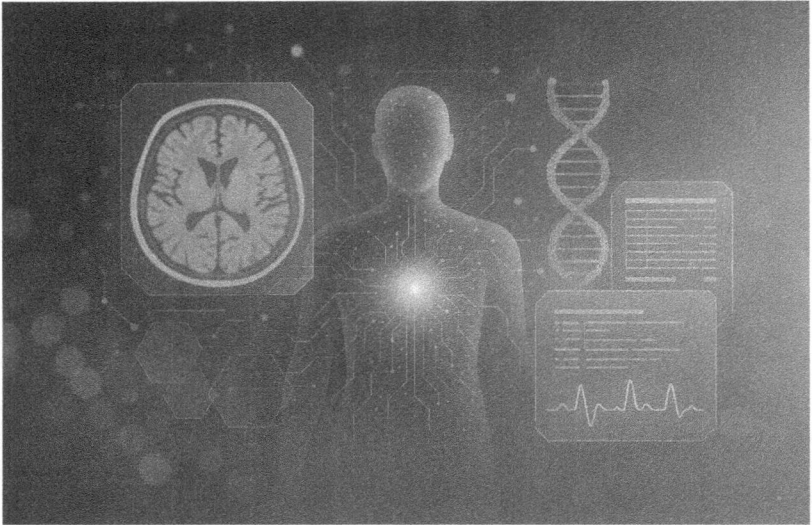

Multimodal models dramatically improve both diagnostic speed and accuracy through sophisticated data analysis capabilities. By simultaneously analyzing diverse medical data types, these systems significantly improve diagnostic insights while reducing the time required for data interpretation. The enhanced diagnostic accuracy results from AI's ability to cross-validate findings across multiple modalities, substantially increasing diagnostic precision and confidence. This improved speed and accuracy enable faster treatment decisions, which directly translates to improved patient treatment outcomes, reduced hospital stays, and more efficient use of healthcare resources throughout the medical care continuum.

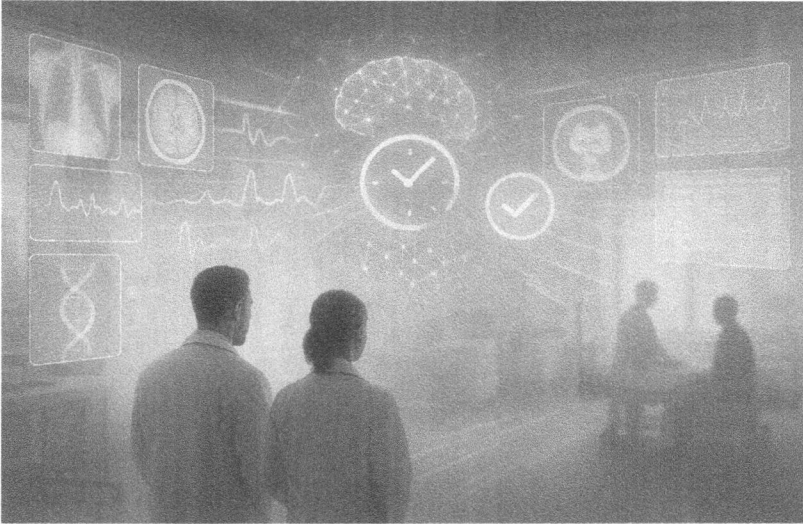

Overcoming challenges in data integration and interoperability remains a significant hurdle for multimodal AI implementation. Heterogeneous data integration requires overcoming complex technical challenges to enable seamless access across different data types and formats. Standardization challenges persist due to the lack of standardized data formats, which impedes interoperability and consistency across various healthcare systems and institutions. Ensuring interoperability between different systems remains vital for effective multimodal AI deployment. Additionally, maintaining high data quality is essential to achieve reliable AI insights and optimal patient outcomes, requiring ongoing attention to data governance and quality assurance protocols.

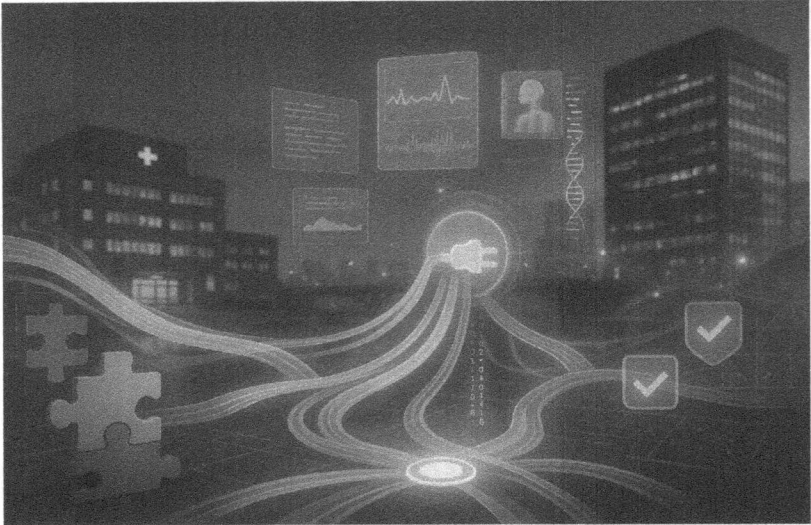

Our final major topic explores AI applications in global health and low-resource settings. This critical area focuses on adapting advanced AI technologies for use in environments with limited computational resources, infrastructure constraints, and reduced technological access. These adaptations are essential for ensuring that AI benefits reach underserved populations worldwide and help address global health disparities.

Adapting AI solutions for resource-limited environments requires careful customization to operate efficiently within significant constraints. AI tools must be specifically customized to function effectively in environments with scarce computational power, limited internet connectivity, and restricted data availability. Infrastructure constraints necessitate adapting AI systems to work reliably within constrained technological infrastructure, ensuring consistent performance and accessibility in underserved regions. Effective adaptation maximizes local impact by enhancing benefits and usability for communities with limited technological access, helping bridge the digital divide in healthcare and ensuring that advanced medical technologies can benefit populations regardless of their economic or geographic circumstances.

AI-driven disease surveillance and outbreak prediction systems provide crucial capabilities for global health security. These sophisticated AI systems analyze real-time health data from multiple sources to detect disease outbreaks early and accurately, often identifying patterns before traditional surveillance methods. Early outbreak detection enables timely responses and effective containment of emerging diseases, protecting public health and preventing widespread transmission. AI facilitates coordinated public health responses by helping allocate resources efficiently and coordinate multi-agency responses during disease outbreaks, ensuring that limited resources are deployed where they can have maximum impact on disease control and prevention efforts.

Bridging healthcare gaps and improving accessibility represents one of AI's most important contributions to global health equity. AI solutions enable scalable and affordable healthcare services that can reach remote and underserved populations previously lacking access to quality medical care. These technologies help reduce healthcare disparities by providing cost-effective AI tools that bridge the significant gap in healthcare quality between well-resourced urban centers and underserved rural communities. By making advanced diagnostic and treatment capabilities more widely available, AI helps democratize access to quality healthcare and addresses some of the most persistent challenges in global health equity.

In conclusion, the future of healthcare AI presents both tremendous opportunities and significant challenges that must be thoughtfully addressed. Innovations including generative models, autonomous agents, and multimodal systems are fundamentally shaping the future of patient care and diagnostics, promising unprecedented improvements in medical outcomes. However, addressing ethical and regulatory challenges remains crucial to ensure safe and responsible AI adoption throughout healthcare systems. The global integration potential of these technologies offers hope for enhancing healthcare accessibility and quality worldwide, but success will require continued collaboration between technologists, healthcare providers, policymakers, and communities to ensure equitable implementation and maximum benefit for all populations.

www.ingramcontent.com/pod-product-compliance
Lightning Source LLC
Chambersburg PA
CBHW050531280326
41933CB00011B/1543